Penguin Books

NOT ON YOUR OWN

Sally Burningham is a freelance journalist who specializes in writing about health and social issues both for the professional press and at a more popular level. After completing a degree in art history at the Courtauld Institute, London University, she worked for some years as an editor in publishing, where she first became interested in the problems of presenting complex ideas in a simple and readable way. While her children were small she acted as a consultant to the National Consumer Council, the Department of the Environment and the then Social Science Research Council on subjects ranging from advice centres and patient satisfaction to planning and ways in which to improve the environment.

Since the mid-1970s her main work has been as a journalist, covering news and conferences and contributing regular features to journals for doctors, social workers, therapists and administrators, as well as to publications for the general reader, especially the parent magazines. A regular monthly column in *Mother and Baby* for three years looked at ways in which parents come to terms with a child's disability and learn to cope. She has also written many health education booklets and reports and contributed to other publications. This is her first book. Sally Burningham lives in Muswell Hill in North London and has two grown-up sons.

Not on Your Own received the prestigious Reckitt and Colman Medical Journalists' Association Award for the most outstanding contribution to medical journalism in 1989.

Sally Burningham

Not on Your Own
The MIND Guide to Mental Health

PENGUIN BOOKS

PENGUIN BOOKS

Published by the Penguin Group
Penguin Books Ltd, 27 Wrights Lane, London W8 5TZ, England
Penguin Books USA Inc., 375 Hudson Street, New York, New York 10014, USA
Penguin Books Australia Ltd, Ringwood, Victoria, Australia
Penguin Books Canada Ltd, 10 Alcorn Avenue, Toronto, Ontario, Canada M4V 3B2
Penguin Books (NZ) Ltd, 182–190 Wairau Road, Auckland 10, New Zealand

Penguin Books Ltd, Registered Offices: Harmondsworth, Middlesex, England

First published 1989
10 9 8 7 6 5 4 3

Copyright © Sally Burningham, 1989
All rights reserved

Printed in England by Clays Ltd, St Ives plc
Filmset in Linotron Melior and Futura

To my parents
with love and thanks

CONTENTS

ACKNOWLEDGEMENTS

So many people have given me such generous help in writing this book that it would be impossible to list them by name. I would simply like to thank them all for their advice and encouragement. Their concern, enthusiasm and openness seemed to me one of the most optimistic signs for the future of mental health.

Though *Not on Your Own* is published in association with MIND, the National Association for Mental Health, the points of view expressed are my own. I would like to thank everyone at MIND for their support, and especially Chris Shaw for reading the text. Thanks also to the Royal College of Psychiatrists for all their help. Finally, a particular thank you to my mother for so patiently commenting on each stage of the manuscript.

INTRODUCTION

We are all likely to experience mental health problems at some time in our life, whether at first hand or as a friend or relative. Yet despite the fact that such problems are so widespread, most of us will feel very much alone when they occur, troubled by what is happening and uncertain what to do for the best. No one should underestimate the distress that such problems can cause. Changed and often unpredictable moods and behaviour are extremely puzzling and upsetting for the people experiencing them as well as for those close to them. However, some of the stress and isolation can be relieved by knowing where to turn for information and support, and by the realization that others have shared the same feelings and experiences.

This book aims to provide clear and simple explanations, information and suggestions to enable people to make the best use of whatever resources are available and choose their own ways to cope. This seems all the more necessary since mental health can be a highly confusing field, even for professionals who work in it. On the one hand there is such a wide range of services, which vary considerably throughout the country both in the extent to which they are provided and in the way they are organized; on the other is the fact that so little is known for certain about mental health problems that people may receive very different explanations and even different advice from different sources. The more information they have, the more they will be able to weigh things up and decide what makes sense for them.

This is not, therefore, a book about solutions to mental health problems. Indeed, there may be none, or not the ones you expect. However, most people have strengths they can draw on, given enough support. Quite often looking for what is still going right in a person's life and building on that is a way forward.

There is no really clear dividing line that indicates when an ordinary difficulty becomes a mental health problem. You will often have to use your own judgement and common sense in deciding whether to seek help for yourself or for someone close to you. Most people accept that a certain amount of unhappiness, anxiety or stress is simply part of normal experience. However, help may be needed if such feelings become overwhelming, if behaviour or attitudes change in a distressing way for no apparent reason or if it becomes harder to cope with ordinary tasks or relationships at home or at work.

Try not to wait for a crisis to develop before seeking help. Problems are much easier to deal with in the early stages. If the person concerned will not talk about the difficulties or go for help, seek advice yourself on how to deal with the situation.

Much of the fear surrounding mental health problems is due to anxiety about coping with unfamiliar situations. One reason people are often unwilling to seek help is because they are unsure of the response they will receive, while friends who might offer support often retreat hastily because they do not understand what is happening and are uncertain as to how to behave. We all need to improve our knowledge of mental health and learn to be more accepting if we are to overcome these anxieties and remove the stigma that is so unfortunately associated with mental health problems.

People who have struggled with mental health problems themselves and those close to them have invaluable expertise to contribute. The more open they can be about their own experience and what helped or hindered them in coping, the more confident, skilled and sensitive we can all become in providing help and support when such problems occur.

This book covers a wide range of mental health topics, including some of the more common mental health problems, the main treatments available, the role of mental health professionals and useful organizations. Confusing mental health terms, current legislation, financial worries and self-help methods are discussed, as well as ways in which friends and relatives can come to terms with their own feelings. It is not necessarily a book you will want to read from cover to cover. You may prefer to select those chapters or parts of a chapter that are most relevant to your needs.

PART I:

PROBLEMS

The following six chapters look at some of the more common mental health problems you may encounter. They are by no means comprehensive. For example, they do not deal with problems related to alcohol or drug abuse or to specific sexual difficulties, all of which are widespread, although useful organizations to contact in these instances are given in Chapter 18.

There are many books written about individual mental health problems. You can ask for suggestions at your local library, from the appropriate organizations (see Chapter 18) or from the professional worker you are seeing. Of course, authors, however balanced, will be putting forward a particular point of view. You may need to read several books to get a full picture of the situation.

It can often come as a relief to be able to put a name to a mental health problem since it helps to make sense of much that has been puzzling. However, it is important to remember that the name is simply an attempt to describe the condition; it is not a label for the person concerned. It is also helpful to realize that mental health problems rarely fit into neat categories. People vary widely in the extent to which they are affected by such problems and in their range of symptoms. Sometimes people are affected by a mixture of problems; it is quite common, for example, to suffer from both depression and anxiety.

CHAPTER 1

Anxiety

The term anxiety can be confusing since it covers such a wide range of experience, from the mild apprehension often felt before an exam to a severe panic attack coming seemingly out of the blue. As a result many people are uncertain as to how much anxiety they should regard as normal and when they should ask for help.

We all feel anxious from time to time. It is simply part of life. Often anxiety serves a useful purpose in helping us to focus our energies on a particular problem or in alerting us to the fact that things are not quite right. If we habitually feel anxious in certain situations, such as speaking in public or preparing a meal for visitors, there are usually self-help measures we can adopt to help us cope. These might include relaxation exercises, practising handling a situation in front of the family or learning to take things step by step.

However, if anxiety should come in some way to dominate your life, either because your reactions are out of all proportion to the apparent cause or because you have an underlying feeling of unease for most of the time, then it is sensible to seek help, initially from your GP (see Chapter 7). It is also sensible to seek help, preferably at an early stage, if your anxiety has resulted in panic attacks, or in phobias, obsessions or rituals which you feel unable to control. You also need to be aware, when consulting your doctor, that anxiety may express itself through physical complaints and that many conditions such as skin rashes, migraine and stomach ulcers, may be partly or mainly caused by anxiety.

Of course there are occasions where you may be extremely anxious for very good reason, such as the serious illness of someone close to you. If this situation and therefore the anxiety are prolonged it is also sensible to see your doctor for support.

Although there is no precise definition of anxiety, we often recognize that we are feeling anxious because of a number of physical, emotional and mental changes that occur, though each of us reacts in our own individual way and according to the degree of anxiety experienced. Among the many physical symptoms that frequently accompany anxiety are stomach churning, shortness of breath, sweating, trembling, dizziness, accelerated heart rate and increased muscle tension. Emotional symptoms may range from feeling frightened or uneasy to feeling restless, tense, unable to concentrate or irritable. Some people may also find that their thoughts dwell on feared situations or possible future events. If anxiety persists for any length of time it can be very exhausting.

No one knows all the causes of anxiety or why some people tend to be more anxious than others but we do know that there are certain situations that are likely to evoke anxiety in many people, and certain attitudes of mind that will foster that anxiety. The more you are aware of your own reactions and take steps to deal with them sensibly, the less likely it is that your anxiety will escalate and become a mental health problem.

Coping with ordinary anxiety

New situations

Many people find that dealing with new situations or unfamiliar surroundings causes some anxiety, though they may be unaware that others feel the same. It is reassuring, therefore, to recognize that it is quite normal to be anxious, for example, when starting a new job, when meeting someone for the first time on whom you want to create a good impression or even when attending a hospital clinic where you are not sure of the procedure.

You may find it helps to talk over your fears with friends beforehand or to rehearse in your mind possible outcomes so that you feel prepared. If you feel very agitated try to sit down somewhere quietly and breathe slowly and regularly for a few minutes to calm yourself. If it is appropriate, admitting openly that you are anxious to those you are with can relieve your tension and enable others to try to put you at ease.

Stress

Stressful situations can lead to anxiety as well as to other mental health problems, though the amount and type of stress that each person can cope with varies considerably. Some people thrive on pressure and deadlines, but taking on too many responsibilities or operating continually against the clock gives rise to tension and anxiety that spill over into all areas of life. Finding the right balance in life is important as too little activity and stimulation can be as stressful as too much.

It may be hard to change a pattern you are accustomed to without support. Talking things over with a sympathetic listener or a trained counsellor (see Chapter 9) might help you sort out your priorities, say no to unwanted demands and allow yourself more time for relaxation.

Lack of appreciation

A lot of anxiety arises when people have a sense of not being in control or not being really needed at work, or at home or in other situations. In such cases it is important that you find other appropriate outlets for your energies and abilities to build up your confidence, such as voluntary work, sport or other activities.

Changes

Changes in life, particularly major changes, are another common cause of anxiety. Most people expect to feel upset and anxious after an event such as the death of someone close, a divorce or a separation, though they may underestimate the length of time it will take them to adapt and come to terms with it. However, they may be less prepared for the anxiety that often accompanies other sorts of change, such as pregnancy, a move to a new home, retirement or even alterations in the routine at work. Recognizing that it is normal to feel anxious about such changes and talking about your feelings, rather than bottling them up, can relieve the strain.

Of course if a number of changes occur close together, the anxiety is likely to be harder to handle. Therefore, where you do have a choice it often makes sense not to move to a new home straight after a bereavement, for example, or to start a new job in the midst of a painful divorce.

Uncertainty

An often unavoidable cause of anxiety is uncertainty. It is obviously quite natural to feel anxious while you are waiting to hear the results of an important examination, whether you have been made redundant or whether someone close to you has a serious illness. If there is nothing you can do to find out more quickly, then keeping as busy as possible and relieving your tension through exercise or relaxation techniques can help to keep your anxiety under control.

Relationships

People usually feel anxious when a relationship seems to be going wrong. When it is difficult to talk it over with the person concerned, it often helps to confide in a trusted friend both to relieve your feelings and to get things into greater perspective. However, if the relationship is a very close one, you may need professional help, as a friend may find it very hard to be objective and to disentangle what is actually happening. If the difficulties involve children, family therapy may be appropriate (see Chapter 10); if they are between partners then Relate: Marriage Guidance could be helpful (see Chapter 18).

Sexual difficulties

Any kind of sexual difficulty can cause anxiety, which may in turn exacerbate the problem. If you are worried about any aspect of sex, consult your GP or the Family Planning Information Service (see Chapter 18), who will offer you information or refer you to an appropriate source of help.

Attitudes

Quite often the attitudes people hold increase their anxieties. Those who tend to be perfectionist and want to excel in all areas are likely to be highly anxious because they have set themselves unrealistic goals. They need to learn to relax their standards and to realize that sometimes it is acceptable to make mistakes. Similarly, those who are trying to please other people all the time, rather than considering what they themselves want from life, are also likely to be anxious since their security rests on the approval of others rather than on their own self-esteem. If these attitudes, or others giving rise to anxiety, are firmly entrenched, some sort of therapy, such

as counselling (see Chapter 9), cognitive therapy or assertiveness training (see Chapter 10), may be useful.

Life-style

Anxiety can be caused or increased by a person's life-style.
Too little exercise, for example, allows tension to build up
in the body, too many caffeine-containing drinks give rise to
anxiety and over-consumption of alcohol will increase anxiety as well as resulting in other problems (see Chapter 12).

Going to your GP

If you go to your GP for help with anxiety or if anxiety is
diagnosed you should not expect a prescription for minor
tranquillizers, except to tide you over a crisis for a few days
(see Chapter 8). Depending on the nature of your anxiety,
your GP is more likely to consider some sort of relaxation
technique, general support, counselling, psychotherapy or a
behaviour-based therapy. You may be referred to a psychiatrist or clinical psychologist for a further opinion and
treatment.

Anxiety often occurs alongside other mental health problems, such as depression, which at the time may seem more
urgently in need of treatment. In that case your GP may feel
that it is more sensible to treat what seems to be the main
problem first in order to see if the anxiety is then alleviated.

Coping with other forms of anxiety

General underlying feelings of anxiety

You may find that you have an underlying feeling of anxiety
for most of the time for no particular reason that you can
identify, or that you are excessively anxious about certain
matters where there is no real need. For example, you might
worry constantly about your financial situation although

you are in fact financially secure, or about the health of your children even when they are perfectly well.

Although these feelings of anxiety may come and go, in some cases they may become intrusive enough to affect your life. They may be accompanied by feelings of apprehension or impending doom or a sense of unreality, as though you are detached and far away from your surroundings, as well as by a range of physical and emotional symptoms, such as those mentioned earlier (see p. 15).

If you are anxious for much of the time, you are likely to be very tense and on edge. Your GP may advise practising some form of relaxation exercise several times a day in order to accustom yourself to relaxing both physically and mentally. People with prolonged and persistent anxiety also tend to adopt fairly negative views of themselves and their environment which, in turn, may tend to reinforce their anxiety. Counselling (see Chapter 9) can help to counter this through building up your self-esteem. Techniques of positive thinking such as cognitive therapy (see Chapter 10) can also help reduce anxiety.

Panic attacks

A panic attack is a period of intense fear or discomfort. It often seems to come out of the blue and usually lasts for several minutes, but sometimes for as long as an hour. The symptoms may include palpitations, faintness or dizziness, excessive sweating, breathing difficulties, choking sensations, flushes or chills, nausea or abdominal upset, tingling, a sense of unreality and a fear of dying or losing control.

Panic attacks can happen to people who are already experiencing recognizable symptoms of anxiety as well as to those who, till then, had not considered that they were particularly anxious. Whatever the situation, a panic attack is especially frightening the first time it occurs and many people visit the doctor worried that there is something seriously wrong with them physically, such as a heart condition. Indeed a series of tests may be needed to exclude the possibility of a physical illness.

Because panic attacks are frequently unpredictable, people often become even more anxious about the possibility of having one at an inconvenient time than about the attack itself, and may restrict their activities accordingly. It is a good idea to consult your GP as soon as you realize you are having panic attacks. Relaxation techniques can usually help people curtail a panic attack when it occurs.

Sometimes some of the symptoms of a panic attack occur because people start to hyperventilate, that is breathe more rapidly and deeply often in reaction to stress. This lowers the level of carbon dioxide in the body, which in turn causes a narrowing of the blood vessels to the brain and reduces the blood flow. The best way to rectify overbreathing is to place a small paper bag over the nose and mouth and breathe in and out. This increases the carbon dioxide in the blood and regulates breathing. Practising slow, regular breathing can also be helpful.

Phobias

Many people experience mild anxiety when confronted by certain objects or situations, but this is very different from a phobia. A phobia is an acute fear that is quite disproportionate to the actual object or situation involved and that cannot be reasoned away even though the person concerned knows perfectly well that their fear is irrational.

People with phobias suffer extreme anxiety and sometimes panic attacks when facing the object or situation they fear. They may also suffer agonies of worry at other times, simply anticipating the possibility of confronting the situation and wondering how they will cope. Fear of fear becomes a further source of anxiety.

In order to escape anxiety as far as possible, most people with phobias try to avoid the situations they fear, although this may considerably restrict their lives. However, it seems that avoiding the feared situation often serves only to increase the anxiety attached to it and further undermines their self-confidence.

The causes of phobias are unclear, though sometimes they develop following an illness or period of stress; at other times, however, they seem to appear for no obvious reason. Only rarely does the anxiety seem linked to a specific event, for example a fear of dogs arising from being attacked by a dog.

The most common phobia among adults seeking help is agoraphobia, a fear of public places. People with agoraphobia may suffer from a wide range of anxieties, including fear of crowds, shops, travelling by public transport, being in a theatre or cinema, walking alone in the street or even leaving home.

A feeling of being able to retreat to a safe place should they feel panic is essential for people with agoraphobia. That is why, for example, if they can visit the cinema a gangway seat is preferable. Travelling by car usually seems to arouse less anxiety than taking a bus or train, as it is generally possible to stop if and when they wish. The presence of a trusted companion in feared situations often provides reassurance.

Another fairly common phobia is social phobia. People with this type of phobia feel highly anxious at the thought of performing certain ordinary activities in front of other people in case they are unable to cope. For example, they may worry about eating in public for fear that they may choke on their food, about writing in case their hand trembles or talking in case they blush or dry up. Or they may have highly exaggerated fears about mixing socially, particularly with the opposite sex.

Then there is a wide range of what are known as simple or specific phobias. These include fear of dogs, snakes, insects, mice, confined spaces (claustrophobia), heights (acrophobia) and air travel.

Sometimes phobias disappear of their own accord after several months, but if they persist for longer and are restricting your life it is important to seek help.

Obsessions and compulsions

Obsessions and compulsions, like phobias, are to do with fears that are recognized as exaggerated and unrealistic by the person concerned, who, nevertheless, seems unable to ignore them. Obsession in this context is not used, as in everyday speech, to mean an infatuation or overwhelming interest, but to describe the insistent recurrence of unwanted thoughts, images or impulses that intrude despite all efforts to resist them.

It is not clear what causes obsessions, but there is no doubt that they can be extremely distressing, particularly, for example, if they take the form of thoughts of harming someone you care about, or fears of causing danger by leaving something crucial undone or repeated blasphemous thoughts if you are very religious.

Sometimes obsessions occur alone and sometimes they give rise to compulsions, or rituals, which may or may not appear to be connected with the obsession. One common obsession, for example, involves the fear of contamination and may result in endless scrubbing and disinfecting a surface each time it is touched. Other common compulsions are excessive handwashing, needless checking and rechecking, and touching various objects in a specific order. These rituals may temporarily relieve feelings of stress, but if they take hold, they will cause even more anxiety as the person concerned becomes unable to manage without them. They may interfere significantly with work, family life or social activities. Rituals can also be very time consuming: often tasks that once took several minutes to complete can take several hours.

Treatment for phobias, obsessions and compulsions

Research suggests that a surprising number of people, perhaps one in twenty, suffer from a restricting phobia or an obsessive-compulsive problem. However, only a minority asks for help; for those who don't, there is the added stress, therefore, of feeling isolated and alone. If you are suffering from one of these conditions do consult your GP. If you would like to talk things over with someone who has a similar disorder you can contact the Phobics Society (see Chapter 18).

Treatment for phobias, obsessions and compulsions is usually based on a variety of behaviour therapy techniques (see Chapter 10) and has proved successful for the majority of people seeking help, providing that they are well motivated, prepared to tolerate a certain amount of distress and to do work at home.

Worries are sometimes expressed that the behaviour therapy approach, which deals only with symptoms and does not involve trying to identify and deal with the causes of the phobias, obsessions or compulsions means anxiety will recur in a different guise. However, this does not usually seem to happen. Far from developing new anxieties, people who overcome their phobias, obsessions or compulsions generally become less anxious and more confident in other areas of their life as well.

CHAPTER 2

Depression

Although more than one in five people are likely to need treatment for depression at some point in their life, there is still a great deal of misunderstanding about the nature of depression and uncertainty about when to seek help. Part of the confusion may be due to the word itself, which encompasses so many shades of meaning from the low mood or passing sadness we all experience from time to time to total black despair.

There have been many attempts to identify more serious, or clinical, depression, as it is sometimes termed, by classifying it into different types (see Chapter 17). However, perhaps the most helpful way to view depression, at least until we have more knowledge, is as a continuum from normal misery to very severe depression, with many stages in between.

Most of us accept that being 'down' or sad on occasion is part of life. These feelings may be due to disappointment, worry or a recent illness, or may arise for no particular reason that we can recognize. Sometimes it can even be a warning that things are not right with some particular aspect of our lives. But as long as these feelings are not too extreme or persistent we usually take them in our stride and are perhaps even motivated to make some positive changes.

However, the situation becomes very different if these feelings are beginning in some way to dominate our lives so that we can no longer cope at work, or at home or with friends, or if they are more severe or long lasting than we might have expected. It is sensible then to seek help from the GP (see Chapter 7) before matters get any worse rather than trying to struggle on.

Unfortunately, many people with depression are reluctant to seek help. This may be because they feel they do not need it, or because they are convinced it will be of little use, or because they are ashamed of not coping. They may need to be reassured by family or friends that consulting a GP for depression is a perfectly sensible and normal course of action. If they cannot be persuaded, then friends or relatives can contact their GP for advice on handling the situation.

Symptoms

There is a wide range of symptoms of depression and any one person is likely to experience only some of them. It is the combination of a number of these symptoms, the length of time they have lasted and the extent of their effect that indicates that the depression has progressed beyond ordinary misery and that some kind of help is needed.

Among the most common symptoms are a predominantly sad, hopeless or irritable mood, a loss of interest or pleasure in all or nearly all activities for most of the time, fatigue and lack of energy, and either a slowing down in both mind and body or increased agitation and restlessness. A high proportion of people with depression also suffer from anxiety.

There may be changes in eating patterns, causing significant weight loss or gain, and changes in sleeping patterns, including difficulties in falling asleep, early morning waking or sleeping longer than usual. There is also likely to be loss of interest in sex. When people are depressed they tend to feel cut off from others, as if there was a barrier round them, and withdraw from social contact, thus further increasing their sense of isolation. They also usually experience difficulty in showing affection, even to people they are fond of.

Problems in concentrating, remembering, or even arriving at a simple decision are also characteristic of depression. So are feelings of low self-esteem, worthlessness, regret, and guilt, often inappropriately directed at some small or imagined incident in the distant past. Very severe depression may sometimes be accompanied by delusions (distorted ideas about the world) or hallucinations (perceptions that others do not share). There may be recurrent thoughts of death or suicide, or even specific suicide plans or attempts.

Sometimes symptoms of depression may be masked by people's behaviour and therefore more difficult to pin-point. For example, some people attempt to deal with their feelings by a frenzy of social activity or by extra work, or turn to drinking for relief, which in turn brings further complications. There are also a great many people who are unaware of their depression, which is expressed through physical complaints such as headaches and other pains. It is often only when the GP has ruled out obvious physical reasons for their condition that they may begin to recognize that they are in fact depressed.

Causes

Most people who suffer from depression are anxious to understand the causes, but though a number of possibilities have been identified, there are, unfortunately, no clear answers at present. However, it seems likely from the research so far that depression is due to a number of different causes and that in many people it is the result of a combination of several interrelated factors, varying from individual to individual.

Stressful and upsetting events, such as a bereavement or divorce, or sudden changes in life-style brought about by illness or unemployment, for example, frequently contribute to a depression. It is, of course, quite natural to feel depressed for a time in such circumstances, but whereas some people manage to come to terms and cope, others for a variety of reasons slip into a more serious depression from which they find it harder to emerge. Sometimes more severe depression develops soon after the distressing occurrence; at other times there may be a delay, often due to not coming to terms with the event at the time it happened.

Anyone can become depressed, whatever their personality, but some people may be more vulnerable than others due to their own individual make-up, or the way in which they have learned to perceive the world, or because of certain early experiences. For example, there is some evidence that adverse experiences in early childhood, such as the loss of a parent, can render people less able to cope with upsetting events in later life and thus more susceptible to depression. It is also likely, but still not certain, that some people inherit a genetic predisposition to depression.

There is some evidence, too, that the circumstances people find themselves in may influence to some extent whether or not they become depressed. If they feel trapped in a situation over which they have no control or are stressed, anxious or lonely and have no one to turn to for support, for example, then depression may well occur. However, it seems that a supportive network of family or friends and in particular a very close, confiding relationship with a partner, relative, or friend can often help to prevent ordinary unhappiness from turning into more serious depression.

The brain is extremely complex but research shows that certain biochemical changes are frequently associated with depression, though whether the biochemical changes cause the depression initially or are caused by it is as yet unclear. However, these changes can often be corrected by treatment with drugs such as antidepressants and the depression lifted (see Chapter 8).

It is known that a number of illnesses and disorders, such as thyroid deficiency and diabetes, can produce depression and that depression may follow certain illnesses such as influenza or glandular fever, even though the person has apparently recovered. It is also recognized that drugs prescribed for certain illnesses sometimes also cause depression as a side-effect. And it is important to remember that alcohol, which people may turn to in order to cheer themselves up, is a depressant, damping down the nervous system; heavy drinking will produce depression as well as other problems.

Almost twice as many women as men admit to depression, but whether this is due to hormonal differences, their situation in life or because they find it easier to talk about depression is not clear. It may be that men bottle up their feelings to a greater extent or are more likely to express them through anger or drinking heavily.

Treatment

Most depressions are self-limiting but untreated they may last many months, or even several years, causing untold misery for the sufferers and those closely involved with them. Early treatment can often prevent depression from worsening and alleviate the symptoms. However, not all treatments work equally well for everyone, and you and your GP will need to find a method of dealing with your depression that is suitable for you. It may be through drugs, or through a talking therapy such as counselling or a combination of the two, or it may involve practical measures such as getting a part-time job, joining a self-help group or taking up a sporting activity. If your depression is caused or exacerbated by difficult living conditions or a low income, your GP may suggest you see a social worker to help you sort out the problems.

If your depression is fairly mild or seems to be related to a particular issue, such as a relationship problem, your GP may decide to see you on a regular basis to talk things over and offer support, or may recommend some form of talking therapy (see Chapter 9). This might be with a counsellor attached to the practice or from a voluntary agency such as Relate (see Chapter 18), or with a private counsellor or psychotherapist. If individual or group psychotherapy is available on the NHS in your area and your GP feels you might benefit, you are likely to be referred first to a consultant psychiatrist (see Chapter 7).

One therapy that has so far proved as effective as drugs in combatting less severe depression is cognitive therapy (see Chapter 10). This aims to convert the negative thought patterns and behaviour that accompany depression into a more positive approach to life. It is not widely practised at present, but it might be worth asking your GP to find out if it is available locally.

If your depression is more severe or has lasted a considerable time, your GP is likely to recommend treatment with antidepressants in order to alleviate the depression itself or to enable you to improve sufficiently to tackle some of the problems contributing to the depression (see Chapter 8). Recent research has shown that the likelihood of depression responding to an antidepressant is not determined by whether or not the depression follows an upsetting life change, but by the severity and duration of the depression.

In other words, the more severe the feelings, the more likely that the depression will be alleviated by antidepressants.

People often worry that antidepressants are addictive. This is not usually so; however, they do need to be administered with care, and, initially, your doctor will need to see you about every two weeks to check the dose and possible side-effects. If one type of antidepressant drug does not prove helpful to you, your doctor might try switching you to another. It is important to remember that the effect of antidepressants takes some time to build up in the body, so you might not start to notice improvements for two or more weeks. It is also crucial to realize that you may need to remain on medication for some months after you feel better to avoid the chance of a relapse.

Unfortunately, about 30 per cent of people with severe depression do not respond to antidepressants. For some others drug treatment may be considered too risky, if they have heart disease for example, or too slow acting if the depression is so severe that they are in danger of harming themselves. In such cases the GP is likely to refer them to a psychiatrist for a further opinion or more specialist help. If the depression still does not respond, or if it is accompanied by delusions or hallucinations, then electroconvulsive therapy (ECT) is likely to be considered (see Chapter 8).

Self-help

There is no one right way of handling depression. You need to find out for yourself what seems to work best for you. However, there are some widely-used self-help measures that may prove helpful.

Talking about your feelings to an understanding listener may bring a sense of relief and can sometimes help to prevent a mild depression from progressing. Sharing feelings with someone who has experienced a similar type of depression and who has come through is also reassuring. Like many people who become depressed, you may be convinced that no one has ever felt quite the way you do before and this can be both worrying and frightening. Contacting a self-help organization for people with depression or a voluntary organization such as the Samaritans (see Chapter 18) can also be a way of overcoming this sense of isolation.

Regular exercise in the open air, such as walking, will help to keep you fit, enable you to sleep better and may alleviate the depression. Eating a sensible, balanced diet will also help you to feel more like coping. Many people go off their food when they are depressed and feel lower than ever because they are missing out on essential nutrients. Though sleep is often disturbed during depression simply resting can be beneficial. Rather than worrying about lost sleep try to find ways of helping yourself to relax such as relaxation exercises. And finally, if you are depressed you should try to avoid drinking alcohol. It acts as a powerful mood depressor and in the long term will make you feel even worse (see Chapter 12).

It is important to accept that when you are depressed you are likely to have far less energy than usual and will therefore be unable to carry out your normal quota of activities either at work or at home. However, it is often helpful to try and do a number of small tasks each day both to keep your mind off the depression and to gain a sense of achievement.

Friends and relatives

If you are a relative or close friend of someone who is depressed, you may feel quite at a loss as to how best to offer support. So often it seems as though the depressed person is giving you a double message of 'I need your help' and 'Keep your distance'; on the one hand being dependent and demanding, and, on the other, rejecting offers of assistance or becoming angry or unfairly critical. It will probably seem to you that the person is behaving in an unbelievably self-centred way and is quite unaware of all the efforts you are making.

It is important to realize that this is part of the depression. Even if you are unable to understand the depth of feeling involved, it may help to remember that the depressed person is even more bewildered, anxious and lonely, and desperately in need of reassurance that things will improve. When people are depressed they often believe that they are quite unlovable, and crave signs of affection and approval, although they may not be able to respond in any way; it is all they can do to cope with their own feelings. Try not to feel hurt if you are rebuffed; it is usually not meant personally, but is anger at the world in general, and your continued support is certainly needed.

Among the most helpful things you can do are simply to listen if the person feels like talking and to show affection in a gentle way if that seems appropriate. If you are not living with the person, then regular phone calls and visits can provide reassurance. You need to resist the temptation to tell them to pull themselves together. If they could, they would have done so, as being depressed involves very unpleasant and painful feelings. Moreover, it is the type of comment that will convince them that you really do not understand.

Depression often causes people to have a distorted view of themselves and the world, so you may find it difficult to persuade your friend or relative that they ought to see a doctor or accept some other form of help. They may suspect that you are trying to manipulate them for your own ends.

Often, suggestions to seek help prove more acceptable when they are made by people who are less close.

Being with someone who is depressed for any length of time can be very draining. It is important to make sure that their depression does not monopolize your life and that you keep up your own interests, otherwise you may start to feel low yourself. You should remember that it is quite normal to feel impatient, irritated and even angry if the depression has been going on a long time. It is vital that you find some support for yourself and some release for your own feelings, perhaps through talking matters over with a good friend.

Bereavement

The death of someone close is for many people one of the most distressing experiences that they will undergo. It is important that they should keep in regular contact with their GP, at least during the year following the bereavement, since they are likely to be in a very vulnerable state both physically and emotionally. They will also need a great deal of support from family and friends, not just in the first few weeks but over several years. The process of mourning and coming to terms takes far longer than many people realize.

It is important that people should be encouraged to grieve and express their feelings rather than putting on a brave front. Those who push their feelings aside and bury themselves in activities often find that they become depressed in later life and have to go through the grieving process then.

How people grieve varies from individual to individual, but there are certain stages that most people pass through. The first is one of shock where the feelings are numbed and the person often appears to be coping, on the surface, particularly with practical matters. However, it is important to realize that they are not in a normal state and try to persuade them not to make major changes, such as moving house.

This stage is often followed by a period of preoccupation with the dead person. The bereaved person seems unable to accept what has happened and waits for the dead person to reappear. Sometimes they are convinced that they have heard the dead person's voice or seen them in the street. They may also feel anger and guilt: anger at doctors, for example, for not doing more to prevent the death or at the dead person for leaving them alone, and guilt at some trivial oversight on their own part. It is during this period that the bereaved person may feel most despairing, depressed and alone. Unfortunately, it is also a time when most friends and relatives expect them to return to normal life. They need to realize that the bereaved person may now have a greater need than ever of comfort and support.

Recovery is often a gradual up and down process. People who have been bereaved are likely to be prone to upset and depression for several years. Low points often come at anniversaries. The GP should always be contacted if the bereaved person seems unable to cope. Support is also available from voluntary organizations such as Cruse-Bereavement Care (see Chapter 18).

Suicide

Most people shy away from the subject of suicide but it may be a very real risk if someone is seriously depressed and you need to be alert to hints and signs. Signs may include complaining of being unable to sleep, becoming very withdrawn and unable to relate, expressing feelings of uselessness and hopelessness, constantly dwelling on problems for which there seem to be no solution, setting their affairs in order or talking about suicide or suicide plans.

It is important always to be prepared to listen if someone

broaches the question of suicide, even if it is introduced in a jokey or off-hand way. It may be upsetting for you but it is often a relief to the person concerned to express their feelings openly. There is no need to feel that you have to counter their arguments or provide solutions. Simply showing that you accept that the person feels as they do at present, though you cannot share their views, and staying with them while they are distressed, can do much to help, at least temporarily.

It is vital never to seem to disbelieve someone who talks of suicide, as this may push them into a 'dare' situation. Moreover, the idea that people who talk about suicide do not attempt it has long since been discredited. If someone is expressing suicidal ideas or conveying that intention in other ways and you feel the matter is urgent, you should try to persuade them to see their doctor immediately. If they are unwilling, you can ring the GP and ask for a home visit. In these circumstances it is always better to err on the side of doing too much rather than too little.

Even if you feel the situation is less urgent, the person's GP should be informed as soon as possible, and it is always a good idea to get support for yourself and advice on handling such a stressful situation. Talk to your own GP or to an agency such as the Samaritans, who have great experience in this field (see Chapter 18).

CHAPTER 3

Manic-depressive Disorder

Manic-depressive disorder is the name given to a condition that is characterized by swings of mood either to mania, a state of abnormal elation and over-activity, or to severe depression, or both. These swings are usually interspersed with periods of relative normality. Of course, many people experience changes of mood ranging from times when they are low and lacking in energy to others when they are more optimistic and full of enthusiasm, but these are usually within manageable bounds. In manic-depressive disorder the swing may be so great that the person concerned is no longer in control of their own actions and medical help is needed.

The fact that manic-depression follows no consistent course can make it harder for sufferers and those close to them to deal with and more difficult for others to understand. For example, while some people regularly experience extremes of both mania and depression, others may find that mania predominates with only mild depression or vice versa, or that the pattern changes over time. Similarly, the frequency and length of episodes vary considerably between individuals and sometimes at different periods of a person's life. Mood swings may be cyclical over a day, a month or a year, for instance, or seem quite random with perhaps several months or many years elapsing between episodes.

What confuses the picture still further for the lay person

is that definitions of the disorder vary. Some doctors diagnose manic-depressive disorder only if an episode of mania, with or without depression, has occurred at some point in the person's life. This is the definition adopted in this chapter. Others prefer a wider definition that includes very severe depression even when there has been no evidence of mania. Severe depression in this context is covered in Chapter 2. These differences are simply over classification; they do not influence treatment. Manic-depressive disorder is also sometimes referred to as bipolar illness.

It appears that manic-depressive disorder affects about one person in 200 to 250 throughout the world, though not all will experience the extremes of the condition. It also occurs more commonly among women. Manic-depressive disorder is rarely diagnosed in children below the age of 14, but it can begin at any time from adolescence on right up into old age. No particular personality type has been associated with the disorder.

Causes

Though there is uncertainty about the causes of manic depression it seems likely that there is a genetic component, at least in some cases. Research suggests that certain people inherit a predisposition to the disorder, which may then be precipitated by other factors at some point in their lives. What these factors are is not completely clear. However, it seems that a highly stressful event may act as a trigger for the illness in some people; in others it may be the hormonal changes that take place at adolescence, childbirth or the menopause. Research also suggests that there is a chemical imbalance in the brain during episodes of manic-depression that affects feelings and behaviour, though its cause is unknown.

Symptoms

There is a wide range of symptoms in both the manic and depressed phases of the disorder. The symptoms vary from person to person, and even in the same person during different episodes, yet another unpredictable factor that makes this condition so hard to come to terms with. Occasionally someone may even experience a mixed state, with symptoms of both mania and depression.

Among the more common symptoms of depression are loss of energy and motivation, lack of interest and pleasure in all or nearly all activities, slowing down of thoughts and physical movements, and a reduced ability to concentrate, remember or make decisions. There may also be a loss of interest in sex, withdrawal from social contact, and anxiety, sometimes accompanied by agitation and restlessness. There may be a marked change in sleeping and eating patterns as well as feelings of sadness, worthlessness and inappropriate guilt, recurrent thoughts of death or suicide and even suicide attempts. It is important that medical help is sought as early as possible before symptoms become too acute.

Many of the symptoms of mania and hypomania (mild mania) are almost the reverse of those of depression. They include greatly increased energy and activity, feelings of elation, excessive self-confidence and lack of self-criticism, and a markedly decreased need for sleep. In the early stages of mania and in mild mania ideas flow rapidly and speech accelerates, often sounding unusually witty or perceptive. In later stages, however, thoughts start to race and speech becomes over-excited, incoherent and incessant. A lowering of inhibitions sometimes leads to a variety of sexual involvements, and loss of judgement can result in disastrous spending sprees, unwise investments or impulsive decisions such as suddenly putting the house up for sale without consulting a partner.

Anger and irritation are easily aroused. During a manic episode people tend to lose their tempers over trifles and become quickly annoyed if others cannot follow their train of thought. They are often highly critical, speak their mind without thinking, and sometimes verbally abusive, even to comparative strangers. Failure to eat proper meals and lack of sleep combined with intense activity often result in exhaustion.

In more extreme forms of mania symptoms, such as unintelligible speech, delusions and hallucinations, are very similar to those occurring in schizophrenia (see Chapter 4); it is then not always easy to distinguish between the two conditions.

Some people are at their most productive and creative during periods of mild mania, benefiting from the increased energy and able to utilize the flood of imaginative ideas that so often characterizes the condition. However, if the mania progresses, they will increasingly lose control and the results can be very destructive both for them and for those who are closely involved with them.

Unfortunately, it is extremely difficult to persuade people experiencing mania that they do need help since in the early stages they feel on top of the world and at later stages they often lose insight into what is happening due to the nature of the condition.

Treatment

Though there is as yet no cure for manic-depressive disorder, mood swings can be controlled or reduced for about 70 to 80 per cent of sufferers through the regular and careful administration of lithium salts (see Chapter 8). In addition to lithium other drugs may also be used. For example, antidepressants are often administered for episodes of severe depression, and major tranquillizers for episodes of mania. For those for whom lithium proves unsuitable or ineffective, the drug carbamezepine may be tried. Electro-convulsive therapy (ECT) may sometimes be used to treat severe depression and very occasionally to treat mania (see Chapter 8).

Early treatment can limit the severity and length of an attack, so persuading someone to visit their GP at an early stage is an advantage. Hospital admission may sometimes be necessary, and it is, of course, preferable if this is on a voluntary basis. However, this may not always be possible during a manic episode as the person concerned is often unable to accept that anything is particularly wrong. Compulsory admission to hospital may occur when it is judged that the person is a danger to themselves or others (see Chapter 16).

Visits to hospital can be very difficult for close friends and relatives, particularly if the person is extremely distressed or accusatory, but they do help to maintain contact and may reassure the sufferer. It is important, therefore, that people should try to keep going regularly, though visits need only be brief.

Normal phases

Most people will return to their normal selves after a bout of mania or depression without suffering any physical after-effects from the illness. However, there are likely to be other problems to come to terms with, such as loss of confidence, anxiety about the possibility of a further attack and regret or embarrassment over behaviour during the illness. Some people may even have to cope with the loss of a job, financial ruin or a broken relationship. It is essential that relatives and close friends rally round during this time to offer affection and support. Though psychotherapy and counselling are not advisable during an episode of mania or severe depression, some form of supportive psychotherapy or counselling during normal periods can assist in restoring confidence and helping people come to terms with their condition.

Friends and relatives

There is no doubt that manic-depressive disorder imposes a very great strain on relatives and close friends, testing their strength, patience and adaptability often to the limit. They may need to assume total responsibility during episodes when the person concerned is not amenable to reason. This could involve measures such as hiding household poisons and tablets, tactfully removing cheque-book and credit cards and managing to mislay car keys, as well as trying to ensure that the person receives appropriate treatment.

Even if they succeed in coping with the hurtful criticism, the deep despair or the exhausting and infuriating behaviour that are all part of the condition, they may have difficulty in switching back to an ordinary give and take relationship once the person recovers. They should realize that they may need considerable support themselves either from friends or a professional counsellor (see Chapter 9) in order to cope with the stress and come to terms with their own feelings.

It is often helpful if ways of dealing with possible future recurrences of the illness can be discussed while the person is well. It may then be possible to agree on measures such as putting the house in joint names or putting affairs in trust to safeguard against impulsive decisions.

Manic-depressive disorder can be as isolating for relatives as for those affected. Talking about the problems associated with the condition can help to relieve the stress. The Manic-

Depression Fellowship self-help groups (see Chapter 18) can give both sufferers and relatives the chance to meet others who have undergone similar experiences and to offer each other mutual support.

CHAPTER 4

Schizophrenia

About one in every hundred people will suffer from schizophrenia at some time in their life. Schizophrenia does not mean split personality (see Chapter 17). Schizophrenia is the name given to a distressing mental illness or group of mental illnesses, in which the different parts of the mind such as thoughts, sensations, memories and emotions no longer function together harmoniously, in the way we normally take for granted, and instead become disintegrated and disordered. As a result the person affected is unable to trust their own reactions and the world becomes a bewildering and often frightening place where fantasy and reality are sometimes indistinguishable.

Schizophrenia occurs equally in men and women, though the age of onset tends to be earlier in men, and across all races and classes. Schizophrenia rarely occurs in children. It makes its first appearance most commonly in adolescence or young adulthood, with the majority of sufferers experiencing their first episode between the ages of 15 and 35, though it can start at any time right up into old age. Its incidence is similar in countries throughout the world.

Causes

It is not yet clear whether schizophrenia is one disorder or several different but closely-related disorders. Nor is it apparent whether there is a single main cause, as yet unidentified, or a variety of contributory causes.

It is evident from research studies that inheritance plays some part, at least in certain instances, since there is an increased risk of schizophrenia for children of a parent who has schizophrenia. About one in ten such children will themselves develop the condition in later life whether they remain with their natural parents or are brought up by other people. New methods of genetic research are being used to try to find out how and why inheritance may contribute to schizophrenia.

One theory, popular in the 1960s, was that certain types of family upbringing could cause schizophrenia. Though now largely discarded due to lack of evidence, the influence of this theory still unfortunately lingers on in some places, sometimes resulting in unnecessary guilt and upset. What has been found to be much more helpful is to concentrate on the important part family and close friends can play once the illness has been identified. It is now widely accepted that calm, undemanding but supportive relationships can assist recovery while a highly emotional, argumentative and tense environment can exacerbate the illness.

It is difficult to be sure what part stress might play in contributing to the onset of schizophrenia. In some people the first episode is preceded by a highly stressful event but in others it seems to occur without there being any obvious stress. However, once people have developed schizophrenia, they become highly susceptible to any form of stress, and pressures, unexpected changes and conflicts can precipitate further attacks.

Symptoms

The onset of schizophrenia may be sudden and dramatic or it may build up slowly, with the person affected gradually

becoming less sociable, less able to concentrate, less affectionate and more withdrawn. If the beginnings are gradual,
they may quite naturally be mistaken for moodiness or, in a
young person, attributed to an adolescent phase.

There is a wide range of symptoms in schizophrenia.
Some of these may be present in various combinations at
any one time or they may occur one after the other at various
stages of the illness. Not all people with schizophrenia
experience exactly the same symptoms, and different symptoms, which may vary in intensity – from the very mild to
the more extreme – may come and go.

Most people with schizophrenia will experience disturbances in thinking, which they will find worrying and upsetting. They may find they are unable to think clearly or order
their thoughts coherently because their mind is overwhelmed with a jumble of ideas or because it suddenly
seems to go blank for no apparent reason. As a result their
speech may seem strange and disconnected and often difficult for other people to make sense of.

Quite frequently people with schizophrenia develop delusions; that is, distorted ideas about what is actually happening. For example, they may believe that someone is inserting
thoughts into their mind, or extracting their thoughts with a
machine or plotting to kill them in a particularly bizarre
way. No amount of rational argument or reassurance will
change these beliefs. Rather than either disagreeing or col-
luding, others often find it helpful simply to say 'Yes, I
understand that is what you believe, although it is not how
I see it.'

Similarly, people with schizophrenia may also be subject
to disturbances of perception or sensation, which are known
as hallucinations. When these occur, people see, hear or
even feel, smell or taste things that other people do not
experience, but which nevertheless seem quite real to them.

One common form of hallucination is to hear imaginary voices coming from inside one's own head or from somewhere else such as the television set. These voices may be friendly or hostile and the person who hears them may hold conversations with them out loud or in their own mind. Sometimes it may appear as though the voices are trying to take control, and this can be very upsetting.

Schizophrenia also affects the emotions in a variety of ways. Sometimes it seems to intensify feelings, so that people are either very miserable or highly excited, or occasionally even violent or suicidal. More often, however, it seems to have a blunting effect, so that people become less responsive and affectionate, and more withdrawn and difficult to make contact with. At times schizophrenia causes people to react quite inappropriately to certain situations, laughing at a sad event or crying at a joke.

Some of the more extreme symptoms of schizophrenia, such as delusions and hallucinations, are often termed florid, or positive symptoms. Though very distressing they usually respond well to treatment, which normally consists of appropriate medication (see Chapter 8) and social support in a calm, stable environment.

A number of other symptoms, sometimes termed negative symptoms, reflect the lack of energy and motivation that is also characteristic of schizophrenia. People may withdraw from social contact because they are so bound up in struggling with their problems and find it less demanding to be on their own. As a consequence they may spend long periods alone in their room sleeping or appearing to do very little. If they do remain in company, they may make little effort to interact and seem quite cut off and self-absorbed. They may also find it hard to concentrate for very long and show little interest in activities, so that holding down a job becomes difficult. Sometimes concern over personal appearance and cleanliness also diminishes.

These negative symptoms may disappear if the person recovers quickly, but if the person is affected over a long period they may become entrenched and much harder to deal with. Unfortunately, negative symptoms do not usually respond to medication. What does seem to be helpful is just the right amount of structure and stimulation in the person's life to awaken their interest without causing stress.

Getting help

People suffering from schizophrenia may be aware that things are not right, but the very nature of the condition means that they may not possess enough insight to understand the kind of help they need. As a result, relatives or close friends may have to persuade them to visit the doctor and accompany them there or, if they are unwilling, contact their doctor for advice. (For help in extreme circumstances see Chapter 16.)

There is no test for schizophrenia and many of the symptoms are similar to those found in other conditions. Delusions and hallucinations, for example, are also symptoms of severe depression and mania and certain drugs such as LSD can produce effects very similar to schizophrenia. If this is the first occurrence of symptoms, a GP is likely to refer the person to a psychiatrist who may, in turn, decide to admit the person to hospital. This will often be in order to determine whether the symptoms are due to schizophrenia or another condition before starting on treatment. If the person is very distressed, then rest and nursing care in hospital may prove beneficial in themselves. Careful questioning of the patient and relatives and observation of the patient's behaviour will assist in the diagnosis. Sometimes people show a mixture of symptoms, so the picture is confusing and a satisfactory diagnosis can be made only after observing the person's response to treatment or after several episodes of illness.

Unfortunately, even when schizophrenia has been diagnosed, it is very hard to predict what course the illness will take and doctors may be unwilling to give an opinion for fear of being too pessimistic or optimistic. Probably about 25 per cent of people who suffer from schizophrenia are likely to have one episode and no recurrence of the illness while about 10 per cent will be seriously affected all their lives. Of those in between, some will manage with only occasional relapses, while others will not recover completely and will require considerable support.

Treatment

Drug treatment, mainly with major tranquillizers (see Chapter 8), enables the majority of people with schizophrenia to live within the community, though they will still require a great deal of social support. Drugs help to control the more acute, positive symptoms, such as delusions and hallucinations, and enable people to think more clearly and generally feel less restless and anxious.

People affected by schizophrenia often lose confidence in interacting socially or in performing everyday activities. A number of different approaches may prove helpful. Social skills training (see Chapter 10) is often suggested, particularly when the person has had schizophrenia for some time or has lost confidence through being in hospital. Regular supportive discussions, including helping the person to adapt to sudden changes, are often beneficial. Supportive work with the family (see Chapter 10) can also be helpful, particularly if the person with schizophrenia is living at home, since there are likely to be problems that everyone will need help in dealing with.

Community care

Organized social support is particularly important for people with schizophrenia whether or not they are living with their family. They need to be in an environment that will make just the right demands on them without exerting too much pressure, and which will encourage greater activity and independence, as well as overcoming their isolation. Unfortunately, however, although about 90 per cent of people with schizophrenia live in the community, such resources are still far too scarce, particularly in view of the policy to close down some large psychiatric hospitals (see Chapter 11). Relatives or close friends should ask social services (see Chapter 18) about day centres, clubs, sheltered workshops and housing schemes. The local MIND group or National Schizophrenia Fellowship group (see Chapter 18) may have further information about what is available in the area and may run their own projects, such as drop-in centres or social clubs.

Family

There is no doubt that living with someone with schizophrenia puts a great strain on the whole family, not least because former methods of relating may no longer be appropriate and new ways have to be learned if distress is to be minimized.

Although the behaviour of the person with schizophrenia may seem very odd and difficult at times and cause a great deal of worry, criticizing, or showing anger or irritation will usually make things worse. Nor will it help to express very natural feelings of anxiety. It seems as though people with schizophrenia only have the energy to cope with their own overwhelming feelings and are unable to handle anyone else's emotions, however reasonable. They will find it far easier to manage if members of the family are able to distance themselves a little and pursue their own interests and activities, while remaining unflustered and supportive.

People with schizophrenia also cope better if they can become more independent and lead their own lives. They should, therefore, be encouraged, where appropriate, to get a job, attend a day centre, or even live separately in a hostel or group home, for example.

If schizophrenia is long-lasting or recovery is not complete, then the family may take some time before they can come to terms with their disappointed expectations. Sometimes the hardest thing to learn to accept is that the person may often be unable to respond to affection, or contribute very much in the way of companionship or even show the family that they are in some way needed. Members of the family are themselves likely to need support in order to cope in the best possible way with this difficult situation. The National Schizophrenia Fellowship (see Chapter 18) has a network of support groups all over the country.

CHAPTER 5

Difficulties in Childhood and Adolescence

When parents worry about their child's well-being or behaviour, they often feel as though their anxieties are unique. It can help to remember that bringing up children is rarely straightforward and that many other parents will have similar concerns.

General worries

There are many different and acceptable ways to bring up children. However, each child is so individual that an approach that works well with one particular child may not be appropriate for another. Although parents usually know their own child best and are generally aware when something is wrong, they are often too close to the situation to understand exactly what is happening and may be at a loss to know what to do for the best. In such cases outside help can often be useful in assisting them to work out what the problem really is and in encouraging them to find suitable ways of handling it.

Children rarely talk about what is troubling them, if indeed they know. Instead they show their distress in a variety of ways that parents often find puzzling and difficult to deal with. They may have inexplicable aches and pains or they may find it hard to manage the next stage of development, such as staying dry at night, going to school or going out with friends. Sometimes they may seem to be slipping back into earlier, more childish behaviour or give signs that all is not well by appearing extremely angry or withdrawn. There may be a particular problem, such as stealing, which gives rise to concern or there may be general behaviour problems at school but not at home, or vice versa.

Any parents who are at all worried about their child at any stage should trust their own instincts and judgement. They may have to be persistent in order to get the support or services they need, but they have a right to talk to a professional who is familiar with the problems of childhood and who can help them make sense of the situation. They should not be put off by people who have little knowledge of children's difficulties labelling them as over-anxious parents or assuring them that their child is just going through a phase.

Sometimes problems do resolve themselves, but it is never a waste of time to talk to an experienced professional, even if simply for reassurance. Moreover, there are many difficulties that can be more satisfactorily tackled in childhood or adolescence, when they first occur, particularly as members of the family are then usually available to help work through the problems and offer support. Problems that are not dealt with at an early stage may well resurface in a different guise in adult life; they are then often harder to resolve as attitudes have become more entrenched.

Sources of help

If you are worried about your child, the first person you will probably consult is your GP, or your health visitor if your child is under 5. Health visitors (see Chapter 7) have a great deal of knowledge and information about young children and can often help you work out an appropriate course of action, particularly with problems such as eating and sleeping difficulties, bed-wetting and temper tantrums. They will, of course, advise you to see the GP if necessary, or can refer you direct to a child guidance clinic, should you wish.

The GP will want to rule out any possible physical cause for the problem before discussing with you what line of action to adopt. Some GPs take a special interest in children and may be able to help you sort out the difficulties if they are not too complex; others may decide to refer you on. Depending on the nature of the problem and who is available in the area, the GP may refer you to a paediatrician – a doctor specializing in the care of children – for problems such as failure to grow or make progress or unexplained aches and pains, or to a child guidance clinic (sometimes called a child and family centre) in the community or to a hospital-based child psychiatric clinic.

If the GP does not suggest it and you feel you need more specialist help, you should ask to be referred. A GP referral is necessary for a paediatrician and usually for a hospital-based child psychiatric clinic. However, in many areas you can refer yourself to a child guidance clinic by letter, telephone or by calling in. You can ask for the address at the doctor's surgery, at your child's school or at the library, or you can look it up in the telephone directory; it should be listed under Education in the entry for your local authority.

Child guidance Hospital-based child psychiatric clinics and child guidance clinics (see also Chapter 10) are staffed by similar teams of professionals and deal with the same type of problems. Whether you are referred to one or the other is usually a matter of convenience.

Members of the team are likely to include a child and adolescent psychiatrist – that is, a doctor with special training in psychiatry and further training in child psychiatry – a clinical psychologist in the hospital clinic and an educational psychologist in the child guidance centre, a social worker and perhaps a child psychotherapist. Each will use their own particular skills and who you see may depend on what the problem is and on who is free, particularly as the service is so stretched.

The first interview is an opportunity for the therapist to listen to what you and your child have to say and to try to assess the situation. Sometimes this assessment may take several sessions. Other close family members may also be invited to attend, as everyone in the family can contribute; each has a different view of the problem and different ideas on how to tackle it.

It is quite normal for parents to feel rather anxious and even guilty when they attend the first session. However, you should not worry that you will in any way be blamed for your child's problems. You should simply try and come in a receptive frame of mind, prepared to think over any suggestions for help that are made and ready to take on board those that seem appropriate, even though this may mean changes in your own attitudes and behaviour.

You should regard this as the time to ask questions about the type of help being offered and the time commitment involved. If you have any reservations or feel that the methods suggested are not suitable for your child, you should talk this over with the therapist at the time; he or she may be able to allay your doubts or discuss whether there are alternative methods of help available.

You should not expect the therapist to provide an instant solution. There may be no easy answer to the problem. The therapist's aim will be to discover, with you, what the best ways of helping your child might be, building on the strengths that your family already possesses.

Family therapy may be offered to your whole family (see Chapter 10), or your child may be offered behaviour therapy (see Chapter 10), group therapy, or individual psychotherapy (see Chapter 9). In individual psychotherapy whatever is discussed between your child and the therapist remains confidential; however, in this instance you would usually be given support as well to help you handle the situation.

If there is a considerable gap between appointments, you should ask how you can get in touch with the therapist should more problems arise.

School If your child has a problem that is likely to be related in some way to school, it makes sense to talk things over first with the class teacher or the year or pastoral head to see what suggestions they may have. Sometimes the school may recommend consulting an educational psychologist (see Chapter 17) from the School Psychological Service, or you might suggest this yourself. In some areas parents can refer themselves to the School Psychological Service (ask your local education authority); however, it should not be seen as a crisis service, so do not wait till matters get out of hand.

The role of the educational psychologist is to give advice and assistance where there are particular worries about a child's progress or behaviour at school or anxieties about school that may be expressed in a variety of ways, including refusal to attend school, sometimes known as school phobia. No child can be seen without parental permission.

The educational psychologist may observe children in the classroom or talk to them on an individual basis to try to establish how they see the problem. You and your child's teachers will be involved in providing information about the child and in helping to devise ways of tackling the problem and seeing that these are carried through. As an objective outsider, the educational psychologist can often help parents and teachers to change their approach and find new and more effective ways of supporting the child, which in turn improve the situation.

An educational welfare officer or educational social worker may be attached to your child's school. You may be put in touch with them through the school to talk over difficulties if your child has not been attending school because of anxieties, prolonged illness or truanting, for example, or if you wish to discuss welfare benefits or referral to other specialist agencies, such as child guidance.

Help for adolescents It may be more difficult to find help for an older adolescent than for a younger child, partly because services for this age group are so sparse and partly because older adolescents generally want to preserve their privacy and may be unwilling to accept help from anyone associated with their parents.

If you are worried, the first step is usually to try to persuade your child to visit the GP. If this is not possible, then you can talk things over with the GP, who may be able to arrange for someone else, such as a social worker, to see your child, thus preserving the child's independence. Alternatively, the GP may refer your child to an adolescent group within the community.

Child guidance and child psychiatric clinics will see children up to school-leaving age, but many older children will be unwilling to accompany their parents. However, in such a case, you can still go on your own to discuss your anxieties about your child. Most clinics will see parents in this way, even if their child has left school.

Some social workers have a great deal of experience in dealing with problems affecting children, particularly adolescents. You can contact a social worker through social services (see Chapter 18) to talk matters over. The social worker may arrange to see your child, if that is appropriate, or put you in touch with other helpful organizations.

There are a number of organizations that provide counselling and drop-in centres specifically for adolescents, though these vary from area to area. There are also a number of voluntary organizations that offer help with particular problems, such as drug abuse and anorexia. Citizens Advice Bureaux, Councils for Voluntary Service and local libraries are useful sources of such information (see Chapter 18). It is often a case of making the best use of what exists.

Specific problems

There are certain problems that parents find particularly hard to identify and deal with, even though they may be aware that all is not well. You need to be alert to inexplicable changes in your child's behaviour and attitudes, and seek help if these are worrying and persistent. Some of these problems are discussed below.

Depression

There is disagreement among professionals as to whether or not depression, as experienced by adults (see Chapter 2), occurs in younger children. There is no doubt, however, that children from a very early age can experience real misery and deep unhappiness. Some ways in which younger children express these feelings are through listlessness, lack of interest in their surroundings or in play, angry or unmanageable behaviour or by becoming accident prone. Of course, there may be other reasons for any of these symptoms, but whatever the cause, it is sensible to seek advice at an early stage.

Recognizing depression in adolescents can be equally

difficult, though for different reasons. Children by this time have usually begun to distance themselves from their parents, who will be less in touch with what is going on in their lives. Moreover, although emotional ups and downs are common at any age, they often appear more pronounced in adolescence and parents may be unsure as to when to intervene. You may need to take some steps if the depression seems to last for more than a few days, if it seems to be a more extreme reaction to an event or disappointment than might have been expected or if there appears to be no obvious cause. Signs to watch for are similar to those in depression experienced by adults and include changes in sleeping and eating patterns, not being able to get up in the morning, staying in their room alone for long periods and withdrawing from friends and other activities. Parents should try, if they can, to talk to their children about their feelings and persuade them to get help. (see pp. 57–8)

Suicide One worry at the back of many parents' minds, if their child becomes depressed, is the possibility of suicide. Suicide attempts are fairly uncommon before adolescence, though they do occur, but the incidence starts to rise steeply during adolescence. Any hint or mention of suicide should always be taken very seriously (see Chapter 2). If your child is unwilling to see the GP, you should talk to the doctor yourself to see what help might be available. If your child has made a suicide attempt, then it is crucial that he or she receives professional support immediately afterwards, either from a psychiatrist or social worker at the hospital, or from an experienced counsellor (see Chapter 9).

Manic-depressive disorder and schizophrenia
Both manic-depressive disorder (see Chapter 3) and schizophrenia (see Chapter 4) may start to develop in the mid-teens. They are usually easier to treat if they can be detected

early. In addition to the symptoms described in Chapters 3 and 4 children may display inexplicable changes in their school performance and in behaviour within the family. Talk over any worries you may have initially with your child's teachers, if he or she is still at school, and with the GP.

Child sexual abuse

This is the cause of a great deal of mental distress at the time it occurs and is likely to give rise to mental health problems in later life if it is not acknowledged at an early stage and help offered there and then. It is, of course, very painful for any parent to discover that their child is being or has been sexually abused, but you should not ignore the possibility if there are physical signs or sudden changes in your child's behaviour that make you suspicious, or if your child drops hints or, indeed, tells you directly. If you are at all worried, you should contact social services (see Chapter 18). It may be distressing to bring this problem out into the open, but it is certain to be more distressing for your child in later years if nothing is done.

Anorexia

Anorexia is an eating disorder that frequently starts in adolescence, often following a period of dieting. Young people with this problem seek to reduce their weight by eating a minimal amount of food and often by exercising strenuously. Even when their weight falls far below the normal level, they remain convinced that they are over-weight. Controlling the amount they are eating becomes an obsession, and restricted food intake means that feelings and perceptions eventually become distorted. Those suffering from anorexia will rarely accept help voluntarily or admit that anything is wrong, and they will often lie and deceive in order to avoid eating more. Your early intervention is essential, as the longer this condition continues the harder it is to deal with, and it can be fatal. You should consult your GP and ask for help from a psychiatrist specializing in anorexia, if necessary.

Bulimia is another eating disorder that may also start in adolescence. It involves the compulsive eating of large amounts of food, often over a short space of time, frequently followed by periods of strict dieting, self-induced vomiting and purging with laxatives to counter the effects of excessive eating. Anorexic Family Aid (see Chapter 18) offers information and advice on anorexia and bulimia.

Children's worries about parents

Parents need to remember that children worry about their well-being just as they worry about their children's. They are aware of tensions and anxieties in your life, even if they are unable to express their concern. If you can explain why you are upset, without becoming too emotional or offloading your problems on to them, it may ease their anxiety. Children often blame themselves for their parents' unhappiness, particularly in the case of a separation or divorce. If you and your partner decide to separate, you should try to be as open as possible about what is happening, while reassuring your children both about practical arrangements and the fact that they are still wanted and loved. Children will naturally be upset, but they will cope far better if they have easy access to both parents and are not pushed into taking sides or obliged to listen to stories of blame. Children often find it a great relief to air worries about their parents to a sympathetic outsider.

CHAPTER 6

Mental Health Problems in Elderly People

Many people regard growing old with trepidation, equating it with failing health, declining mental powers, loneliness and misery. But this is, in fact, far too pessimistic a picture. The vast majority of elderly people are independent, active and alert and often as happy and contented as at any other time in their lives. Of course, this is not to say that people are not vulnerable to a range of mental health problems in old age, just as at any other time of life. Two of the main mental health problems that affect people in old age, and which give rise to a great deal of concern, are depression and dementia.

Depression

Depression is discussed in general terms in Chapter 2. Unfortunately, depression in elderly people all too often remains unrecognized and therefore untreated. This may be for a variety of reasons. For instance, many elderly people live alone, and friends and relatives who see them only from time to time may fail to pick up the signs. Elderly people tend more often to complain quite strongly of the physical symptoms associated with depression, such as aches and pains, rather than of feeling low, so that even doctors are sometimes misled into searching for physical remedies rather than identifying depression. Finally, many people seem to believe that it is quite normal for elderly people to appear sad, particularly if they are approaching the end of their lives. It is important to remember that the quality of life counts at every age. There is no reason why elderly people should accept feeling depressed, since nearly all depression can be successfully treated.

Some of the causes of depression are described in Chapter 2. Physical ill health and disability are particularly common factors in depression among elderly people. So too is bereavement. The effects of certain drugs, either on their own or in combination, are also significant in contributing to depression, confusion and forgetfulness in elderly people who are more likely to take a number of drugs for a variety of ailments, and who are more susceptible to their effects because of their slower rate of metabolism. The doctor might therefore decide to see whether reducing the number of drugs taken or cutting down the dose is beneficial.

Some of the symptoms of depression, such as loss of appetite, should be taken particularly seriously in elderly people, who are often physically more vulnerable. Failure to eat properly is likely to be a risk to health. Symptoms such as agitation, lack of concentration and failure of memory are often particularly distressing to elderly people and difficult to distinguish from the confusion associated with dementia. An early diagnosis is therefore important so that appropriate help can be given.

Friends and relatives

The best help you can give to an elderly friend or relative who you think may be depressed is to persuade them to see the doctor and talk things over. You could also contact the GP yourself to supply additional helpful information, if possible with the person's permission.

Your support will play a crucial part in their recovery

whether the doctor decides on medication or other forms of treatment. You should try to dissuade the depressed person from making any major decision, such as entering residential care or moving in permanently with a relative, while they are still low, as they may later regret it. As the depression begins to lift, you may be able to look at some underlying problems with the person concerned, such as lack of day-to-day contact with other people or lack of an enjoyable activity. You can contact social services and voluntary organizations (see Chapter 18) to find out what resources exist in the area.

Dementia

Dementia is the general term for a number of brain disorders in which an irreversible decline in mental functioning takes place including the loss of the ability to think, reason or remember. The likelihood of developing dementia increases as people get older. It is relatively uncommon below the age of 65, affects perhaps between 2 to 3 per cent of the population between the ages of 65 and 75 and possibly as many as 20 per cent of those over the age of 85.

About half those people suffering from dementia have a condition known as Alzheimer's Disease. It is named after the German neurologist who described the abnormal brain changes that occur in this condition and which can only be seen under a microscope. It is not yet clear what causes Alzheimer's Disease or why some people should develop it rather than others. It occurs equally across all groups in society and is not related to stress or whether the person has led a highly active or inactive mental life. According to recent research inheritance is likely to play a part, at least in a small number of cases. Alzheimer's Disease is terminal, although some sufferers survive ten years or more.

Multi-infarct dementia, sometimes known as cerebrovascular or arteriosclerotic dementia, probably accounts for a further fifth of people with dementia. It occurs when a series of small strokes take place within the brain itself and damage areas of the brain. Multi-infarct dementia is more common among those with a history of high blood pressure, circulatory problems or other major strokes. Unlike Alzheimer's, where deterioration is steady and gradual, multi-infarct dementia progresses in a step-like way. The person will deteriorate after each stroke and then remain on a plateau, or even improve slightly, until the next stroke.

Approximately another fifth of people with dementia suffer from a mixture of Alzheimer's and multi-infarct dementia, while the remainder are due to a number of rare conditions, not all identified.

Diagnosis

So far there is no medical test for dementia. Diagnosis is usually made by excluding the possibility of other conditions that have similar symptoms such as confusion, forgetfulness, restlessness and agitation. Most of these conditions are treatable so it is important to contact a doctor straight away when someone starts to behave in a confused manner, giving relevant background details such as a recent illness or change in circumstances as well as when the confusion was first noted, to aid the doctor in the diagnosis.

Among the various causes of confusion, apart from dementia, are depression, as already described, infections, particularly chest or urinary infections, infected leg ulcers or pressure sores, thyroid gland deficiency, vitamin deficiency, too much medication or even relatively small amounts of alcohol. Confusion in the elderly can also be caused by a sudden alteration in surroundings or a major upset such as a bereavement.

The diagnosis of dementia will come as a shock if you are a close friend or relative since there is no known cure. However, at least it will enable you to make sense of extremely puzzling behaviour and to start to come to terms with the situation. The sooner help and support can be organized, the better for everyone.

Each person with dementia will react in their own individual way and decline may take place over a number of months or years. However, many people with dementia will experience similar kinds of problems. That is why it can be so helpful for you to talk to professionals in the field and to other carers at an early stage.

Course of the illness

Dementia normally begins very gradually. You might be aware that something is not quite right with another person, perhaps even for a year or so, but find it hard to pin-point. They might seem more apathetic or indecisive than previously or more irritable or easily agitated. They are likely to be forgetful, particularly of recent events, and slower to grasp ideas. Behaviour often becomes more self centred and less concerned with others.

As dementia progresses changes become more marked and the person concerned will need a great deal more help in managing day-to-day living. You may notice that they become confused about the time or day or where they are or forget the names of friends or close family members or even mix people up. More worryingly they might turn on the gas and forget to light it or leave saucepans to boil dry on the cooker.

Some people behave very inappropriately, for example going out in their nightwear, or become active at night when everyone else is sleeping or wander from the house on their own and become lost. You may find that you have to encourage the person to wash and eat regular meals, or help with dressing and other routine tasks. Communication is likely to become increasingly difficult, perhaps because the person repeats the same remark or question time and again or is unable to find the right word or understand more complex sentences. People with dementia usually become very easily upset. Sometimes they may even seem to have changed personality, becoming more aggressive and suspicious or very anxious and tearful.

In the later stages of dementia the person is likely to become totally dependent on others for care. Their speech may make little sense and they may lose the ability to understand others. Most distressing of all is that they may no longer recognize even those closest to them.

Help and support

Unfortunately, there is as yet no treatment which will halt the decline which occurs in dementia. However, certain measures can be taken to help prevent its acceleration, such as keeping the person physically fit through regular meals, exercise and prompt treatment of any physical ailments. Emotional upsets and sudden changes in environment can also cause deterioration. People respond better to a quiet, familiar routine although carers need support and regular breaks. Introducing the person to other helpers and to new settings, such as a day centre, at an early stage in the illness, enables them gradually to accustom themselves before they become too confused.

Many of the carers of people with dementia are themselves elderly and need to take particular care of their own health, if they are to be able to continue with the exhausting task of caring. It is important that they and other carers make full use of any help and support available. The GP is the first point of contact both for help and advice on how to cope and for access to other services such as the district nurse, the community psychiatric nurse, occupational therapist, and continence adviser or for referral to a hospital specialist, day hospital or respite care. Social services (see Chapter 18) are another important initial contact for services such as home helps, meals on wheels, incontinence laundry, aids and adaptations and respite care. Many voluntary organizations also offer information, practical assistance and support. Ask about voluntary services at your local Citizens Advice Bureau, Council for Voluntary Service or local Age Concern or Alzheimer's Disease Society group (see Chapter 18).

Looking after someome with dementia is often very distressing and many carers develop mental health problems of their own. It is vital that carers make sure that they have time to themselves to relax and lead their own life in order to safeguard their mental health. It is also crucial that they have the opportunity to express their bottled-up feelings to an understanding listener.

One common emotion experienced by carers, at different stages of the illness, is grief at the gradual loss of the person they used to know. Carers also frequently feel guilty, either because they believe that they are not doing enough or because at times they resent the task of caring and perhaps even wish that the person were dead. At other times they may simply feel angry at having to carry such a load, embarrassed by the person's behaviour or puzzled how best to cope with the change in roles if a parent or partner becomes totally dependent. Self-help and support groups, which may be run from the local hospital or surgery or by the Alzheimer's Disease Society, provide an opportunity for carers to unburden themselves, share their experiences and overcome their isolation.

There is no one way to handle someone with dementia. Each person is different and the situation may well be changing all the time. If you are a carer you will need to find out by trial and error what works best for you. Generally speaking, the more flexible you can be, the better.

It is important to allow people to do things for themselves whenever possible, even if it takes much longer, and to let them help you with routine tasks while they can in order to keep them active and to preserve their dignity. As communication becomes more difficult, try to speak in simple sentences dealing with one point at a time. Try also to be encouraging if they are having problems finding a word or finishing a sentence.

People with dementia respond best to a calm, relaxed approach. This is not always easy, as you are probably under considerable stress, but if you can find ways to relax, both of you will benefit. Showing affection is also a way of remaining close. Simply sitting holding someone's hand, putting your arm round them or giving them a hug are all ways of maintaining contact and reassuring them that you care.

PART II:

PROFESSIONAL HELP

The following five chapters describe the main treatments available for mental health problems, the role of the mental health professional and hospital care.

Because the causes of many mental health problems are complex and not entirely understood, it is not always clear which treatments, or therapies as they are sometimes termed, will be helpful for which individual. Sometimes a doctor may try a number of treatments in turn or suggest that the problems may best be tackled by a combination of treatments; you yourself might also ask about the possibility of trying a particular treatment.

Physical treatments include the use of drugs and electro-convulsive therapy (ECT). In the talking and behaviour-based therapies the person being treated plays a far more active role. Unfortunately, the availability of both talking and behaviour-based therapies throughout the country is patchy, but if you feel that a particular therapy might be useful to you, it is worth asking your doctor about it. Even if it is not offered locally, it may be available elsewhere if you are prepared to travel.

It is easy for both patients and relatives to pin unrealistic hopes on a particular treatment and expect rapid major improvements. Some therapies do seem to work quickly for some people, but often recovery – if it does take place – is a slow process. Although uncertainty is very hard to cope with, you will probably find it more manageable if there is a time limit. It makes sense, therefore, to ask your doctor or other mental health professional approximately how long it might be before you could expect some improvement, however small, to take place. If no such change occurs, you should certainly discuss alternative approaches. Of course, sometimes you might have to accept that the situation will not alter greatly. Part of the treatment may consist of helping you to come to terms with this and adjusting your expectations accordingly.

Some therapies may be offered privately, but do take care. Anyone can use the title counsellor or psychotherapist or, indeed, any other sort of therapist. Even a row of certificates on the wall does not prove that they have the skill and training needed to help you work through your problems. Ask your doctor, psychiatrist or someone whose judgement you trust to recommend a properly trained therapist or suitable organization for you to contact. If you do go privately, make sure you check on charges before you start, as these can vary considerably. Some therapists have a fixed fee; others operate a sliding scale depending on what you can afford.

People often become upset and defensive if some form of talking or behaviour-based therapy is suggested. They feel it indicates that something must be very wrong with them. In fact, everyone could probably benefit from some kind of therapy, as we all have areas in our lives where we feel confused or function less effectively. Therapy gives us the opportunity to sort out these areas and many people find that it gives them an added strength. However, in order to benefit you need to be prepared to work hard and be very honest with yourself. Perhaps, most important of all, you must want to change.

CHAPTER 7

Professionals in the Mental Health Field

If you seek help with a mental health problem or because you are feeling very distressed, you are likely to encounter members of one or more of the professions described in this chapter. Professionals in the mental health field often work as a team or in close consultation with each other, and their roles may frequently overlap. Which person you see most of may well depend on the arrangements in your particular area.

Most mental health problems are complex, and different professional workers may concentrate on different aspects, depending on their skills and training. Often it is not possible to tackle all aspects of a problem, but sometimes support in one area may help you to feel strong enough to deal with other parts of the problem yourself.

One common failing among professional workers is the tendency to talk in jargon, assuming everyone will understand them. Never be afraid to ask them to explain themselves in everyday language. It is not your task to master their specialist terms and theories; it is their responsibility to make themselves clear.

Another frequent shortcoming among those in the mental health professions is the tendency to offer explanations with such authority that they sound like certainties rather than the suggestions they usually are. This can be particularly confusing if you find yourself offered quite different explanations with apparently equal conviction by practitioners in different fields or even by practitioners within the same field. You need to remember that many mental health problems are still not fully understood and that these explanations are just different ways of looking at a problem and shedding light on it, which may or may not prove helpful in your particular case.

Be as open as you can but if, after thinking carefully about any explanation or suggestion you are offered, it does not seem to ring true for you, say so and why, so that you and the person you are consulting can begin to look at other possibilities. After all, professionals do not have magic insights; they can only base their knowledge of you on what you tell them and what they can observe.

There may be times when you are unlucky and encounter professional workers who seem intent on fitting you into a theory rather than listening to what you say and seeing you as an individual. Just be aware that this can occasionally happen, and try not to let it upset you too much. Your own common sense should prevail and, if necessary, you should seek help elsewhere.

If your customs and background are very different from the professional worker you are seeing you need to be aware that this could give rise to difficulties. People in this country come from a wide variety of ethnic, social and cultural backgrounds. Certain beliefs and ways of expressing emotion which are entirely acceptable within one community may sometimes be misunderstood by a professional worker from a different background and inappropriate help or treatment offered as a result. Of course, professionals should make every effort to increase their knowledge of different groups in society, but this is bound to be a gradual process. If you feel that such difficulties might occur when you consult a professional, particularly if you are not fluent in English, make sure you take someone with you from your family or community who is articulate and can help to put your problem in perspective.

When you first seek professional help for a mental health problem, either for yourself or someone close to you, you are probably hoping for an immediate solution and are likely to feel let down if you discover that none exists. However, even in these instances professional workers have an important role to play. They may be able to help you adjust to a new situation or find a better way of coping. Most importantly of all, they may be able to help you tap your own strengths and resources, which you had not realized you possessed.

General practitioner

The vast majority of patients with mental health problems are treated by their GP. Your GP should be your first port of call whenever such problems are suspected. If you are feeling very anxious or depressed, or otherwise unable to cope, or if your behaviour has changed in a worrying way for no obvious reason, then do consult your doctor. The sooner your problem can be identified, the sooner appropriate support or treatment can be offered and the less distress it is likely to cause you and your family.

Some people are very reluctant to talk to their doctors about emotional or psychological problems because they assume that it is the GP's task to deal only with physical illness. However, between a quarter and a third of a GP's patients come for help with problems such as anxiety or depression or have illnesses with a strong psychological component.

If you as a relative are very worried about someone close to you who will not visit the doctor you could ring their doctor yourself and explain your anxieties. It is often a relief simply to talk and the doctor may be able to suggest means of help, depending on the circumstances. Remember, however, that though the doctor can listen and ask questions, he or she will not be able to discuss the person with you in detail, since that would be a breach of confidentiality.

Of course, our minds and bodies interact so closely that sometimes it is hard to determine what is due to physical illness and what to mental stress. That is why your doctor may wish to give you a physical examination and perhaps some tests if you complain of a problem such as depression. He or she may first need to check whether there is an obvious physical cause for the way you are feeling – such as an illness or the aftermath of one, the side-effects of any drugs you are taking, or even an inadequate diet – before going on to discuss other possible reasons.

Similarly, your doctor will be well aware that many people express anxiety, depression or stress through physical symptoms. If no physical cause can be found for your backache or migraine, for instance, it would be sensible for you and your doctor to consider whether emotional tensions may be playing a part.

You will obviously need more time to talk to your doctor about the way you are feeling than you usually would about a routine physical complaint. If there is an appointments system, you could try booking a double appointment. If not, and your doctor seems harassed because the surgery is full, ask if you can come back for a longer session. If you find it hard to talk about yourself or feel very nervous, there is nothing to stop you writing to your doctor to explain your situation, as you see it, before the appointment. You could also take some notes in with you to jog your memory, or ask a friend or relative to accompany you.

Your doctor will probably want to ask you a number of questions about your feelings and about whether you or anyone in your family have experienced psychological difficulties before; this is to try to determine what the problem might be and what kind of help might best be offered. You should tell the doctor about any particular stresses in your life, and any significant changes in your behaviour; for example, in the way you relate to other people, in your sleeping and eating patterns or in your work. Try to be as open as you can. Sometimes it may be helpful for your doctor to talk to a close friend or relative, but this would only take place with your consent.

Your doctor will not be able to come up with a solution for every mental health problem. Sometimes it may be a matter of coming to terms with things as they are, or trying out a variety of common-sense approaches and seeing which helps the most, or just visiting the surgery for a regular chat until things improve. There is often no one right way to tackle a problem, and different GPs may prefer different approaches, depending on their interests, their experience and the different facilities available to them.

You should never be afraid to ask your doctor about alternatives to methods suggested or ways in which you might be able to help yourself. You might inquire what is available in the area in the way of counselling, for example, if that seems appropriate, whether there are any useful self-help groups or supportive organizations, whether you might be eligible for any practical support or whether taking a relaxation class might be helpful. If your doctor suggests prescribing drugs, make sure you ask the relevant questions (see Chapter 8).

Obviously it is important that your doctor is someone you feel you can talk to; some doctors are more interested in mental health problems than others. If you feel that this is an area in which your doctor is not at ease, you could ask whether there is someone else you could talk to in the practice. If this is not possible and you really find your doctor unhelpful, you might consider changing doctors, particularly if you think you are going to need support for a considerable time (see Chapter 18).

If you have a complaint about your doctor, try to sort it out on a personal level first. The doctor may not have realized there was a problem or that you were particularly upset. If you can't sort it out and you want to make a complaint, get advice on the correct procedure from your local Community Health Council (England and Wales), local Health Board (Scotland) or local Health and Social Services Board (Northern Ireland) since making a complaint can be quite complex. The relevant addresses will be in the telephone directory.

Sometimes your doctor may refer you to a psychiatrist or you yourself may ask to be referred. This might be for help in reaching a diagnosis, or because the psychiatrist can offer a wider range of treatment or support.

Psychiatrist

A psychiatrist is a qualified medical doctor who has subsequently completed a number of years of specialist training in diagnosing and treating mental health problems. General psychiatrists see patients with a great variety of mental health problems, although they might also have special expertise in particular fields, such as eating disorders or addiction. Some psychiatrists specialize further in certain areas, such as child and adolescent psychiatry and the psychiatry of old age. Others have further training in psychotherapy and are known as consultant psychotherapists.

Consultant psychiatrists hold senior hospital posts, though they may also work in the community, and they have overall responsibility for the assessment and treatment of patients in their care. However, they usually work in close consultation with other professional staff, such as nurses, psychologists and social workers, in a team, drawing on their observations, skills, knowledge and experience as appropriate. They also work closely with other doctors who are in various stages of training in psychiatry. Though you will be referred to a consultant, you may be seen by one of these doctors, who will then discuss your case with the consultant.

Except in certain cases of emergency and where there are walk-in clinics, you will need to be referred by your GP in order to see a psychiatrist. The appointment will normally be in the out-patients department at your district general or psychiatric hospital, though some psychiatrists hold sessions in doctors' surgeries or community health centres. They may also make home visits, usually in the case of elderly patients.

Unless it is urgent, there may be a wait of some weeks before your appointment. You should telephone and let the hospital know at once if you can't attend so that another appointment can be made as soon as possible. If you feel that the wait is too long, tell your GP, who may be able to bring it forward.

People are often very anxious about seeing a psychiatrist for the first time because they have no idea what to expect. In fact, the interview, which will probably last about an hour, is usually very straightforward. It is important to remember the psychiatrist may have no information about you apart from what is contained in your doctor's letter. He or she will therefore be trying to build up as full a picture as possible of the sort of person you are and the kind of life you usually lead, as well as assessing how your distress or illness is affecting you now. This will help not just in diagnosing what might be wrong, but also in selecting the form of treatment that may be most appropriate in your particular case.

Depending on the circumstances, you may be given a physical examination or certain physical tests. Like the GP, the psychiatrist will want to rule out the possibility of an obvious physical reason for the way you are feeling.

You are bound to be asked a number of fairly straightforward questions about your background and present situation. These are likely to include questions about your upbringing and schooling, for example, your work, family and personal relationships, as well as your medical history. You may be asked about any recent changes you have noticed in your own behaviour, for instance in your eating and sleeping patterns, your ability to concentrate and your general level of energy. You will probably also be asked if you are taking any drugs, whether prescribed, over the counter or illicit, as well as the amount of alcohol you drink.

Most importantly, the psychiatrist will want to find out how you are feeling. This could be rather painful and distressing, or even embarrassing at first, but the psychiatrist is used to hearing people express their feelings, and will try to put you at your ease. Try to be as open as you can.

You might be asked to bring along a close friend or relative because it can be helpful for the psychiatrist to talk to someone who knows you well. Of course, this would happen only with your permission. The psychiatrist might ask a social worker to talk to other members of your family if you agree.

At the end of the interview the psychiatrist will discuss with you the diagnosis and treatment, and this is the time for you to ask questions, particularly about the aims of the treatment. You might see the psychiatrist again for more sessions or another member of the team, such as a clinical psychologist, or go back to your GP for treatment. The psychiatrist will write to your GP.

If it is felt that you need more intensive treatment and support, it might be suggested that you attend a day hospital. If for any reason you are quite unable to cope, the psychiatrist may recommend that you come into hospital for a period of time (see Chapter 11).

Clinical psychologist

If you are depressed, anxious, lacking in confidence or suffering from phobias or obsessions, for example, your GP or psychiatrist may suggest you see a clinical psychologist. You should not be put off by the name. A clinical psychologist is simply someone who has a degree in psychology – the scientific study of human and animal behaviour – and further training in the health field. Their skills are particularly useful in the assessment and treatment of certain emotional and psychological problems.

Careful assessment is considered to be very important so you should not be surprised if your first interview with a clinical psychologist takes quite a long time and you are asked a number of very detailed questions. He or she may also want to interview members of your family, though only with your consent, of course. The aim is to find out exactly what the problem is and how you and others are affected by it before deciding on appropriate treatment.

If your problem relates to anxiety, the psychologist may sometimes carry out certain simple, painless physical tests such as measuring heart rate, sweat rate or muscle tension, all of which may be affected by anxiety. Sometimes, to help in the assessment, you might be asked to carry out observations at home. For example, you may be asked to record the level of your anxiety at different times in the day, or in different circumstances on a scale of one to ten.

Clinical psychologists possess a range of skills and techniques including those associated with both behaviour therapy and psychotherapy or counselling (see Chapters 9 and 10). Treatment, which is geared to meet your needs, may involve a number of skills and you may be expected to do quite a lot of practice at home. Your family and friends can often be very helpful here.

You will probably see the clinical psychologist on a regular basis of perhaps once a week, for a limited period of, for example, three months, though in some cases treatment does last longer. You may also see a clinical psychologist for family or group therapy (see Chapters 9 and 10). Clinical psychologists also work alongside psychiatrists as part of a multidisciplinary team in helping patients diagnosed with more severe mental conditions such as schizophrenia and manic depressive disorder.

Depending on the practice in your health authority you can be referred to a clinical psychologist by your GP, by a psychiatrist or by another professional such as a social worker. In some districts you can refer yourself. If you think it might be helpful to see a clinical psychologist check with your local Community Health Council (see Chapter 18) as to the procedure in your health authority.

Nurses

Nurses in psychiatric hospitals and units known as registered mental nurses (RMNs) have completed a special three-year psychiatric nursing training and have wide experience of many different forms of mental illness and distress. They are sometimes called psychiatric nurses.

These nurses have a wide range of responsibilities and

work closely with psychiatrists and other professional staff. Because they spend so much time with patients their observations are particularly valuable when treatment is being discussed. Many RMNs have had further training and have acquired additional skills; they may carry out individual, group or behaviour therapy with patients (see Chapters 9 and 10).

A state-enrolled nurse who has completed a two-year training with a more practical emphasis in a psychiatric hospital or unit is sometimes referred to as an SEN(M).

Most people find nurses approachable and it certainly makes sense for patients and relatives to talk over any practical problems with the nurse first, whether these are about visiting, upset children, financial worries or how to cope with a weekend at home. If the nurse is unable to advise, he or she can suggest who you should talk to.

Community Psychiatric Nurses

Psychiatric nurses who work in the community are known as community psychiatric nurses (CPNs). All CPNs are registered mental nurses and many have had extra training in community psychiatric nursing. Some CPNs are attached to psychiatric hospitals or units, and others may work from GP surgeries or community mental health centres. Their work includes helping former patients to adjust to life in the community, supporting people with mental health problems who remain at home, organizing support groups and providing therapy. Some CPNs specialize in problems such as drug addiction and alcoholism.

CPNs often carry out assessments of people with mental health problems in their own homes, which can be particularly helpful for elderly people. If you feel that it might be helpful for you or someone in your family to talk to a CPN, ask your Community Health Council (see Chapter 18) what system operates in your area. Depending on where you live, you may be able to approach a CPN directly, or you may need a referral from your GP or consultant psychiatrist.

Health visitor

Health visitors are nurses who have undergone further specialist training in order to offer people advice and information on health care, often in their own homes. Health visitors do not carry out nursing tasks.

Every child under 5 has a health visitor, who makes contact soon after the child is born. Health visitors are available to help parents sort out any worries over the physical health and development of this age group, as well as any emotional problems which may occur such as feeding difficulties, temper tantrums or jealousy of a new baby.

Health visitors are also concerned with the well-being of the whole family and can offer emotional support over matters such as post-natal depression, relationship stresses or anxieties over an elderly relative, as well as practical suggestions on how to cope. They can supply information on local services and organizations and advise on benefits. Some health visitors are particularly skilled in bereavement counselling or in aiding people who wish to come off tranquillizers.

If you are caring for a relative with mental health problems, or have mental health problems yourself and want an opportunity to talk over emotional and practical difficulties, you can get in touch with a health visitor, who may be able to visit you in your home to offer information and support. You can contact a health visitor through your GP, the local health centre or local child health clinic. Local health centres and clinics are listed in the telephone directory under the name of your district health authority.

Some health visitors also run Well Woman clinics, which offer women the opportunity to talk about their health and feelings, as well as providing a physical check-up. Many women find it a relief to admit to depression, perhaps for the first time, or to know that worries over matters such as pre-menstrual tension and the menopause will be taken seriously. To find out if a Well Woman clinic exists in your area, contact your Community Health Council (see Chapter 18) or ask your health visitor.

Social worker

If you or someone in your family has a mental health problem social workers may be able to assist you in two different ways (see also Chapter 18). Firstly, they can offer information and advice on practical matters such as day care, accommodation and benefits, which may lift some of your worries. Secondly, they can look at the problem itself in the context of the family and the community. By talking to everyone who is closely involved, they can build up a picture of how each person is affected and how they respond. They may then be able to suggest alternative ways of handling situations so that they become less stressful for all concerned.

All social services departments will have social workers who are particularly experienced in helping people who have difficulties associated with mental health. Some social workers will work quite intensively with individuals or families to support them through mental health crises.

If you or a relative are in a psychiatric hospital or unit, or attending a day hospital, you can ask to see the hospital social worker to discuss any worries you have about employment, housing, finance or family problems, for example, and how best to cope at a practical level once you or your relative are discharged.

The role of the Approved Social Worker/Mental Health Officer is described in Chapter 16.

Occupational therapist

You are likely to come into contact with an occupational therapist, often referred to as an OT, if you are a patient in a psychiatric unit or hospital or attending a day hospital. The OT's aim is to help you acquire or practise skills that will enable you to become more confident and independent in the outside world.

These may be everyday, practical skills, such as cooking simple meals, doing the washing or going shopping, tasks that may seem rather daunting if you are feeling fairly anxious or distressed, but which you will probably find much easier to manage with some support, guidance and encouragement. The OT may also work with you on social skills such as answering the telephone, inviting a friend for coffee or handling a job interview.

People who have been feeling low or anxious for some time often find that they have lost confidence and that this makes it more difficult to communicate. OTs can help by organizing groups where people can practise on each other what to say or how to handle certain situations, and support each other in tackling real life situations.

OTs also work in the community. They can often help in finding work or other suitable activities for people who have experienced mental health problems.

The OT will often want to talk to relatives and to encourage them to be supportive without being over-protective. Relatives will usually be advised to try to let the person do as much for themselves as they can, even if this takes much longer. OTs can be particularly helpful if you have an elderly relative with mental health problems, since their training spans both physical disability and mental illness.

OTs are employed by both social services and the health authority. Arrangements vary in different areas. If you would like to talk to an OT, contact social services or ask your GP or the hospital.

CHAPTER 8

Physical Treatments

Drugs

If you are considered to have a serious mental illness nowadays, it is likely that medication will form some part of your treatment. A number of useful drugs have become available since the 1950s. Though not providing cures, they have, in many instances, been able to alleviate symptoms in a variety of distressing mental illnesses; they have also made it possible for many people to live in the community rather than remain in hospital.

However, drugs are not a magic solution. Though often very beneficial, they are not necessarily effective in all cases. Moreover, they cannot, of course, solve the problems that contribute to mental illness; in addition they do have side-effects, although these will vary from individual to individual.

If your doctor suggests prescribing a drug for you or a close relative with mental illness, you should spend some time talking it over first. The more you understand about the aims of a particular drug, its advantages and disadvantages and how it works, the more you will be able to contribute to your own treatment or that of a friend or relative. You are less likely to be swayed by the opinions of well-meaning friends or acquaintances, who may not understand the particular problems that are being taken into account.

Most people forget much of what they are told once they leave the surgery, probably because they are, quite naturally, feeling anxious. It can be helpful to have a pencil and paper with you to note down information. You can check up on any details about the drug you may be unsure of with your pharmacist.

The first point to discuss with the doctor is what the aims of the drug are and how important drug treatment is in your particular case. You will want to know whether there are any effective alternative treatments or other treatments that could be used at the same time. If you agree that drug treatment is appropriate, you may have a number of detailed questions about the drug concerned, if your doctor has not already supplied that information.

You will, of course, need to know the name of the drug and whether this is the generic name – that is, the name agreed by an international authority – or a manufacturer's brand name. You will also need to know whether it belongs to a group of drugs, such as antidepressants or major tranquillizers, for example.

You must know how often to take the drug, whether before or after meals, as well as what to do if you forget a dose. It is also important to ask how long it is likely to be before the drug takes effect. Some drugs take two to three weeks, and people who do not realize this may give up too soon in the belief that the drug is not working. You will also need to find out which symptoms the drug should relieve so that you can make some assessment of how well it is working in order to discuss this point with your doctor.

It is also useful to know the more common side-effects of the drug. Some doctors feel that discussing side-effects worries people unnecessarily, since not everyone will be affected in the same way. Moreover, some symptoms that occur after treatment may be due to the condition itself.

However, many people find that they are far less anxious if they know that their slight dizziness or dry mouth, for example, may be due to the drug or the course of the illness rather than to a separate condition. If you do experience side-effects that worry you or are particularly troublesome, tell your doctor about them as soon as possible. Any serious or long-term side-effects also need to be understood so that you can contact your doctor at the first sign.

If your doctor does not mention it, remember to check what effect the drug might have on your general reactions. Will you be able to drive a car or operate machinery, for example? Can you drink alcohol when you are taking the drug, and are there any other foods, drinks or medicine you should cut down on or avoid?

Other drugs, including over-the-counter remedies, may interact adversely with the drug you are prescribed, so tell your doctor if you are taking other medication, even if it is just the occasional aspirin or cough syrup. Mixing certain drugs can be dangerous and, in any case, the fewer drugs you are taking at any one time the better.

Although you will want to know how long you will have to take the drug that has been prescribed you should not be surprised if your doctor cannot give you a definite answer. Each person reacts differently to medication and your doctor will need some time to see how you progress.

Your doctor is likely to check your medical history before prescribing. Mention any points that may have been missed, such as suspected allergies, for example. Always tell your doctor if you think you may be pregnant or are hoping to become so, since, when possible, it is wise to avoid taking drugs during pregnancy.

If you are elderly, you will probably need a much lower dose of a drug than a younger person. Side-effects tend to be more pronounced among elderly people, but less obvious because they are often mistaken for signs of old age. If you have any doubt about the effects of a drug on yourself or an elderly relative, alert the doctor immediately. The dose may well be too high or there may be adverse reactions because of other drugs that are being taken for other conditions.

Remember that if you are prescribed drugs for mental illness you must take them regularly for them to be effective. They will need careful monitoring to get the dose exactly right, so you will need to visit your doctor fairly frequently, at least at the onset of treatment. This will give you the opportunity to discuss any side-effects and air any worries you have about the treatment.

You should never alter the dose or come off drugs suddenly without consulting your doctor. Even if you have made up your mind that you want to stop taking your drugs, you will probably need to do so gradually, under the supervision of your doctor where possible, in order to avoid very distressing withdrawal effects. These can occur even with drugs that are not addictive. Your doctor will also want to keep an eye on you after you have finished taking the drugs to make sure that you are coping well and that there are no signs of a relapse.

Finally, it is absolutely vital to remember to keep all drugs in a safe place well out of the reach of children.

Minor tranquillizers and sleeping pills

Minor tranquillizers and sleeping pills belonging to the benzodiazepine group of drugs were very widely prescribed until the early 1980s for a wide range of anxieties and sleeping problems. Such drugs – often better known by their brand names, such as Valium, Librium, Mogadon and Dalmane – were also frequently prescribed on a long-term basis. However, doctors nowadays are generally far more cautious.

This is because it is now known that these drugs tend to lose their effectiveness at relieving symptoms after quite a short period and that there is a considerable risk that those taking them will become addicted.

Tranquillizers – also known as anxiolytics or anti-anxiety drugs – may be helpful in getting you through a few days of acute or unexpected stress, but they should not usually be taken to alleviate longer term or more deep-seated anxiety. If you and your doctor decide that you need tranquillizers, you should not expect a prescription for more than a week's supply. If your condition has not improved at the end of that period, you need to go back to your GP and discuss alternative ways of tackling your problems.

You should also be aware that tranquillizers, besides making you feel calmer, will slow down your reactions and make it harder to concentrate. They should not be taken if you are going to drive or to operate dangerous machinery. It is important not to drink alcohol if you are taking either tranquillizers or sleeping pills, as the combination will increase the effects of both.

Sleeping pills, like tranquillizers, should usually be taken only as a short-term measure for a few nights if you desperately need some sleep in order to cope. If you have a longer term problem with sleeping, then you need to discuss the possible causes with your doctor. If you are suffering from mild tension, for example, then a simple measure such as a bath or a walk before bed can sometimes do the trick (see Chapter 12). If you are taking sleeping pills make sure that you do not leave them by the bed. It is all too easy to wake in the night and reach out, forgetting that you have already taken one.

Of course, you may be still taking tranquillizers or sleeping pills regularly because you were prescribed them on a long-term basis some time ago, before their shortcomings as drugs were understood. If so, and you want to come off, you should do so very gradually under the guidance of your doctor, whenever possible. If you have become dependent on these drugs, you will also need a great deal of support from friends and relatives when you start to come off. Try to keep active with plenty of not-too-demanding tasks. A tranquillizer self-help group can be very useful. Ask your GP if one exists near you, or contact Tranx, the regional branch of MIND, the Scottish Association for Mental Health or the Northern Ireland Association for Mental Health (see Chapter 18).

Antidepressants

If you have a fairly severe or persistent depression, particularly one with a number of symptoms such as disturbed sleeping or eating patterns, weight change, loss of energy, slowed reactions and feelings of guilt and hopelessness, then your doctor is likely to recommend a course of antidepressants. These drugs cannot solve the problems that may have contributed to the depression, but they can frequently relieve the symptoms and restore you to a state of health in which you are better able to cope. This is of benefit not only to you but also to those close to you.

If you have reservations about taking antidepressants, talk them over carefully with your doctor rather than simply throwing away the prescription or failing to finish the course. There may be alternative ways of helping you that you will find more acceptable or you may decide that antidepressants are a sensible treatment for you once you understand more about how they work.

Incidentally, antidepressants do not help people who simply feel unhappy or miserable and they are not often prescribed for mild depression, since this usually responds better to talking and other forms of support.

Tricyclics The antidepressant prescribed is most likely to be one from a group of drugs known as the tricyclics, so-called because their chemical structure contains three rings of atoms. Sometimes an antidepressant from a group of similar drugs with four rings, known as tetracyclics, is prescribed.

Your doctor is likely to start you on a low dose, which will gradually be increased. This helps to minimize possible side-effects. The doctor will probably ask you to return for a visit every two weeks or so at first so that he or she can monitor the effects of the drug and adjust the dose to suit your needs.

Many people are disappointed because they expect an immediate improvement when they start taking antidepressants but in fact these drugs take some time to build up in the body and it might be between two and four weeks before you start to feel better. Usually physical symptoms improve first. You may begin to sleep better and regain your appetite, for example. Then you may gradually become more alert and active, and find it easier to concentrate and remember things. Finally, your mood should lift, though you may still have the odd bad day for a time.

However, you should not stop taking antidepressants as soon as you feel better, although this is tempting, as there is a strong chance that you may then have a relapse. You will probably be advised to remain on antidepressants for several months longer to be on the safe side and then to come off them gradually. Antidepressants might be prescribed long term for a minority of people who suffer from very frequent bouts of serious depression. If you are one of these people, you should discuss the advantages and disadvantages of such treatment very carefully with your doctor.

Unlike tranquillizers, antidepressants are not addictive, but, like all drugs, they do have side-effects. Among the most common are drowsiness, blurred vision, dry mouth and constipation. Side-effects tend to vary from person to person and usually diminish as treatment proceeds. However, if you find any side-effects very troubling, tell your doctor, who may vary your dose or try you on a slightly different drug. You should avoid drinking alcohol, as this can react badly with the medication.

A major drawback of antidepressants is that they can be used to overdose. Seriously depressed people, who might be contemplating suicide, should be given only a very limited supply; alternatively, a relative or friend could take charge of the drugs.

MAOIs Most depressions respond to tricyclics, but if yours does not or you cannot tolerate the side-effects, your doctor may suggest trying a drug from another group of antidepressants known as monoamine oxidase inhibitors, or MAOIs. These can be very useful where the symptoms of depression include a tendency to overeat or oversleep, or where the person is very lethargic or highly anxious. However, MAOIs have a great disadvantage in that they interact adversely with certain foods with a high tyramine content, such as Marmite and some cheeses, and certain other drugs, sometimes causing a dangerous rise in blood pressure. If you are prescribed MAOIs make sure you have a list of these substances, so that you can take care to avoid them.

Although antidepressants are helpful in alleviating fairly severe depression in more than 70 per cent of cases, they do not seem to be effective for the remainder, for reasons not yet understood. Unfortunately, there is no way of telling in advance who will respond. If you are among those who do not respond to antidepressants, your doctor may advise a course of electroconvulsive therapy (ECT) (see page 100).

Major tranquillizers

The major tranquillizers are a group of drugs used to treat the symptoms of what are sometimes termed psychotic illnesses; that is, conditions such as schizophrenia and mania where the person is very seriously distressed. However, despite being called major tranquillizers, they have nothing in common with the benzodiazepine group of drugs known as minor tranquillizers, which are sometimes prescribed for anxiety (see pp 91–3). They differ completely in their chemistry, their side-effects and almost all their effects. You may also hear major tranquillizers referred to as antipsychotic agents or neuroleptics.

It is not clearly understood how major tranquillizers work, but they do seem to be able to control distressing symptoms such as thought disturbance and hallucinations in many people, and enable them to cope better with everyday living. However, they are not a cure and those who are prescribed them will still need other forms of support.

There is no doubt that the introduction of these drugs in the late 1950s has been of great benefit for many people who would otherwise have spent much of their lives in hospital. However, major tranquillizers do have considerable disadvantages because of their side-effects, some of which are relatively minor and some more serious. Not everyone will experience troubling side-effects but if you do, discuss them with your doctor. It may be possible to adjust your dose or switch to a different drug. In the end it might be that you will have to weigh up the advantages of the drug in controlling distressing symptoms against the drawbacks of the side-effects.

Among common side-effects that you may experience are drowsiness, dry mouth, trembling hands, blurred vision and lowered blood pressure. Some users develop a condition known as Parkinsonism, in which muscles stiffen and weaken, hands shake and movement becomes difficult, though this can usually be reversed by altering the dose. Other drugs can be prescribed to counter Parkinsonism, but they may have side-effects of their own and should be used with caution.

If high doses of tranquillizers are taken for long periods, there can be a danger of damage to the central nervous system. This can result in a condition known as tardive dyskinesia, in which people develop involuntary movements of the face and other parts of the body. You and your family need to be on the alert for early signs of this condition, such as continued blinking and facial twitches.

If you are being treated with a major tranquillizer, you may find it will be some days or even weeks before you begin to experience improvement. As you start to recover, the dose will probably be lowered. Your doctor will probably want you to continue taking the drug for some time after you feel better to avoid the danger of a relapse and then to come off it gradually. Even after you come off the drug you will need careful monitoring. The effects of major tranquillizers remain in the body for some time, so if the drug has been helping, relapses may not occur until several months after you stop taking it. Some people who suffer from recurrent bouts of schizophrenia are kept on a low maintenance dose for several years, and sometimes even for life, as a preventive measure.

Most people take major tranquillizers as tablets or capsules, but long-lasting injections on a weekly or monthly basis are available for people who might be forgetful about taking the drug.

Lithium

If you have suffered from several bouts of mania or mania and depression (see Chapter 3) your doctor may suggest putting you on lithium as a maintenance therapy to try and prevent future episodes or at least reduce their frequency and severity. Lithium, a mineral element that is found naturally in rocks and also in very small quantities in the body, is prescribed in the form of a salt as either lithium carbonate or lithium citrate, though you may be more familiar with it under one of its brand names such as Priadel or Camcolit.

Although we do not understand how it works, lithium does seem to be very effective in stabilizing mood for 70 to 80 per cent of those who suffer from manic-depressive disorder, although unfortunately it does not seem to work for the remainder. However, approximately half of those who do respond and who continue with the treatment experience no more attacks; the remainder are helped, often to a considerable degree. Moreover, though it is frequently prescribed long term or for life, lithium does not appear to be addictive or lose its effectiveness. Anyone prescribed lithium as a preventive measure does need to realize that it may take many weeks before it starts to work.

As well as being used as a preventive measure lithium may also be prescribed to control mild attacks of mania, known as hypomania. In such a case it usually proves effective within five to eight days, sometimes less. However, sometimes in hypomania and usually in more severe attacks of mania a major tranquillizer is prescribed initially since its effects are more rapid. Lithium is also sometimes prescribed for depression. Some depressive illnesses which do not appear to be affected by treatment with antidepressants alone, respond more quickly when lithium is added to the treatment.

Lithium is clearly a beneficial and effective treatment for many people as it appears to stabilize mood without interfering with normal intellectual functioning or the capacity for ordinary emotions such as happiness and sadness. However, it needs to be administered with great care. The margin between a dose that is too low to be effective and one which is high enough to be toxic is far narrower than for many drugs and varies with each individual. Patients on lithium will need to have the lithium level in their blood measured every week at first, and then gradually less frequently once the correct dose for them has been determined. Once the blood lithium level has been established it usually remains very constant except in the case of physical illness, hot, sweaty conditions or a salt-free diet.

Before prescribing lithium your doctor will want to look carefully at your medical history and will need to make various tests. Lithium has to be avoided or used with great caution for people who have some form of heart or kidney disease and in pregnant women, particularly in the early months. It is not prescribed where there is illness involving disturbance of fluid or salt balance. Lithium does not mix well with certain drugs, such as diuretics or anti-rheumatic pain-relieving drugs. If your doctor is prescribing lithium and you are taking one of these medications, he or she will need to monitor you extremely carefully to avoid a toxic overdosage.

Your doctor will also want to ensure that you are eating a balanced diet containing normal amounts of salt and drinking sufficient fluids. Too little salt and dehydration could cause a dangerous build up of lithium in the body.

You may suffer from side-effects from lithium at the onset of treatment such as nausea, vomiting, mild hand tremor or diarrhoea. Tell your doctor about these and any other unusual symptoms. They can usually be avoided by adjusting or retiming the dose. Some people on lithium experience increased thirst and urination after several months. If this occurs inform your doctor. Others may experience considerable weight gain. If this happens to you cut down on sugary and fatty foods but on no account fast or cut down on salt and fluid. Lithium can affect both kidney and thyroid functioning so regular checks are important. It may also sometimes affect fine movement as in handwriting or playing a musical instrument.

It is crucial that anyone who is on lithium is aware of the signs that it may have reached a dangerous level in the body. If you experience weakness, unusual clumsiness in your hands, wobbling unsteadily on your feet, slurred speech and difficulty in thinking clearly, stop taking lithium and contact your doctor immediately. There may be other reasons for your responses but it is better to be safe.

Electroconvulsive therapy

Electroconvulsive therapy, or ECT, is most frequently recommended for people with severe depression who have failed to respond to antidepressants. It is also sometimes a treatment of first choice for depressed patients for whom drugs might be too hazardous, such as people with heart disease, for example, or for those who are so severely depressed by the time they come for treatment that their lives are in danger. Improvements from ECT are generally much faster than from antidepressants. In addition ECT is very occasionally used for people suffering from acute schizophrenia or acute mania who are not responding to drugs.

ECT is regarded with distrust by many people, perhaps due to the crudeness of its early methods and its former widespread indiscriminate use. However, techniques for administering ECT have improved greatly since the early years. It is now a much safer treatment with fewer side-effects. It is also now used much more selectively.

No one quite understands how ECT works but it does

seem to be effective in relieving severe depression in the majority of cases. Patients are given a short-acting general anaesthetic and a muscle relaxant. Two electrodes are attached to the head and a very mild electric current is passed into the brain causing a minor convulsion. The muscle-relaxant reduces the effect of the convulsion to not much more than a twitch.

People will need to rest for one or two hours when they come round and they may experience side-effects such as a headache, drowsiness, dizziness or stiff muscles or muscle pain for an hour or so. However, the main side-effect that seems to worry people most is memory disturbance. Sometimes there may be difficulty in remembering information acquired just before the treatment, and sometimes in remembering information acquired just after the treatment. People are likely to feel less anxious if they are warned that there may be some memory impairment in the short term but that it should quickly right itself. Some people do complain that they have suffered longer term memory loss but it is not clear whether this is due to ECT or to other causes.

There are no set number of treatments in a course of ECT as each person responds individually. However, most people will probably have between 6 and 12 sessions at the rate of two or three a week, either as in-patients or out-patients. Patients may feel better just after a session at the start of treatment and then be disappointed because they have slipped back. It is important to understand that the effects of ECT build up gradually. Most patients find that their depression has greatly improved within a month or so although there is a minority – perhaps about 15 to 20 per cent of those treated – who do not respond at all.

If a course of ECT is suggested for you, you will obviously want to think it over carefully. You should be given the opportunity to discuss the procedure, the possible side-effects and the likely advantages before you make up your mind. If you are a voluntary patient, treatment will not be given without your consent. If you are a detained patient your consent is still required. However, if you refuse and the doctor in charge of your case considers that such treatment is essential, you may still be given treatment in certain circumstances. Very occasionally you may also be given treatment without your consent as an emergency measure (see p. 105).

Studies show that although in some cases ECT does seem to be very distressing, most people who have experienced it find it neither unpleasant nor frightening. Of course, it is also important to take into account that in some cases it may be life saving.

Psychosurgery

Psychosurgery is a treatment for severe, intractable depressive illness and sometimes for crippling obsessional states. It is considered only when all other forms of therapy have failed and the situation is desperate, when perhaps, for example, the patient is making repeated suicide attempts. In fact only about twenty operations a year are carried out in the UK.

Psychosurgery today has little in common with the operation known as pre-frontal leucotomy, or lobotomy, which tended to be carried out fairly indiscriminately in the late 1930s to early 1950s, partly because of the lack of other available treatments. Operating methods were far cruder then and the risk of side-effects, with some patients reduced to almost total passivity as a result of the operation, would be considered quite unacceptable today.

Psychosurgery is now far more precise, patients are far more carefully selected and the risk of side-effects is far lower. The most common method of psychosurgery in this country is to implant small radioactive rods in the brain while the patient is under general anaesthetic. These rods destroy tiny amounts of tissue in very specific areas and become inactive after a few days.

No one yet understands how psychosurgery works but about 60 per cent of people recover sufficiently after the operation to lead an active, normal life while a further 20 per cent experience limited improvement. The remaining 20 per cent show very little change.

The operation does not appear to cause any alteration to the patient's personality except in so far as it returns to the pre-depressed state, nor in the ability to experience emotion. There is, however, a very slight risk of epilepsy developing though this can usually be controlled. It may take several months after the operation for improvements to take place although suicidal feelings may be reduced in a week or so.

No patients ever undergo psychosurgery against their will. Firstly they and their relatives have the opportunity to discuss all the pros and cons with the doctors and other members of staff concerned with the case before they reach a decision. Then, if they are accepted as suitable the operation still has to be approved by a panel appointed by the Mental Health Act Commission under Section 57 of the Mental Health Act 1983 even if the patient is not compulsorily detained. The three independent people on this panel, including a doctor, must certify that the patient has understood the treatment and consented to it. The doctor must further certify that the treatment is likely to be beneficial in this particular case.

Consent to treatment

Unless you are a formal patient detained under certain sections of the Mental Health Act 1983 (see Chapter 16), the doctor treating you – whether a GP or a hospital doctor – must obtain your consent to whatever treatment is proposed.

For your consent to be considered legally valid, should the question arise, it must be shown that you have been given information on the nature and purpose of the treatment, and on any serious side-effects. It must also be shown that you have understood this information and that your consent to treatment has been freely given without you having been pressurized. Moreover, you can withdraw your consent at any time.

In many cases your consent can be inferred from your actions, such as holding out your arm for an injection, or accepting a prescription; this is called implied consent. For some treatments, however, your consent may be sought by asking you to give an express verbal consent to treatment or to sign a consent form. No one else can consent to treatment on your behalf.

Consent to treatment should be sought from children under 16, providing they are mature enough to understand the implications of the decision being made. If you are the parent or guardian of a child who is too young or too confused to give consent, then you may give consent on their behalf. For further information contact the Children's Legal Centre (address on p. 208).

The exception to all this is a case of emergency, where prompt action may be necessary to save someone's life, or to prevent serious danger to the person or to others. In this case treatment can be given without consent simply to bring the emergency to an end.

Of course, in practice some people are too ill or confused to give consent to treatment. In that case, every effort should be made to consult relatives and other professionals involved in their care as to the best course of action.

Sometimes a second independent doctor may be called in to give an opinion on the proposed treatment.

Detained patients

Patients compulsorily detained under the Mental Health Act 1983 for seventy-two hours or less, under guardianship, or remanded in hospital for a medical report, have the same rights to refuse treatment as voluntary patients and those in the community. However, patients detained under other sections (see Chapter 16) can in certain circumstances be given treatment without their consent. For example, they can be given drugs without their consent for up to three months following the initial administration, if their doctor feels this is necessary. After that time, the patient must either give legally valid consent, or an independent doctor – appointed by the Mental Health Act Commission – must decide whether the treatment is appropriate. Before reaching a decision this doctor must consult two people concerned with the patient's treatment, one of whom must be a nurse and one neither a nurse nor a doctor. Patients can also be given ECT without their consent, should this be thought necessary, providing an independent doctor appointed by the Mental Health Act Commission agrees, after following the same process of consultation.

Detained patients can also be treated in case of emergency without consent and without the need for a second opinion but only when it is thought that treatment is immediately necessary to save the patient's life, to stop the patient's condition from seriously deteriorating, to alleviate serious suffering or to prevent the patient from being a danger to him or herself or to others.

CHAPTER 9

Talking Therapies

Just talking through one's problems with an understanding friend is often a great relief; but sometimes this is not enough. We need a skilled and objective outsider to help us sort out our jumbled thoughts and confused feelings. Friends, quite naturally, want to reassure us and find solutions rather than dwell on what is troubling us. They are often too involved to hear clearly what we are saying, and because we know it is hard for them to witness our distress we may tend to disguise how bad we really feel or decide that we cannot bother them yet again.

If you are feeling very distressed, then the first step is to recognize this and share your real feelings with someone outside your immediate circle who is experienced in listening to problems and handling them, and who will not be shocked or upset by what you say. The most obvious person to talk to is your GP, but it might be to a psychiatrist, if your GP refers you, a social worker, someone from your place of worship, if that seems appropriate, or someone on a telephone helpline.

It may be that a number of such discussions with a detached but perceptive and caring outsider, who can give you the opportunity to express your real feelings, is enough support to see you through. But you may decide, having started to look at your feelings, that you need help on a more concentrated and regular basis, and that some form of counselling, psychotherapy or group therapy might be appropriate. Talking therapies can be useful for a wide range of problems, including some forms of depression and anxiety, relationship difficulties, addictions, general feelings that life has lost its meaning, and low self-esteem.

All talking therapies have a great deal in common. They encourage and support people to look closely at themselves and at the links between various parts of their life so that the real nature of their problems and their feelings become clearer, and their positive qualities, too, become more apparent. This may not always solve the difficulties, but it can make them easier to handle and give people a new sense of energy and confidence.

Which talking therapy you select may depend on what your GP or psychiatrist advises, what is available or what feels right for you.

Individual counselling and psychotherapy

There are a variety of different trainings for counsellors and psychotherapists and as some counsellors are also trained psychotherapists, the distinction between the two is not always clear. Quite often their roles also overlap but generally speaking, you might expect a counsellor to concentrate on what is happening in your life at the present and on helping you to sort out thoughts and feelings that lie fairly near the surface. You will, of course, refer back to the past in counselling, but quite often this is simply to shed light on a present-day problem.

In psychotherapy, on the other hand, you might expect to explore the past at least as much, and sometimes more than, the present. Psychotherapy is based on the belief that the roots of many of our problems lie in early childhood experience. Such an approach is sometimes referred to as psychodynamic. This simply means drawing on the past to understand the conflicts of the present. By talking to the psychotherapist about your past and by trying to get in touch with memories and feelings that lie just beneath the surface, you will hope to get closer to understanding some of the underlying causes of your distress. (For an explanation of psychoanalysis, see Chapter 17.)

There is very little free counselling available. Though a few organizations offer free counselling and some GPs have a counsellor attached to the surgery whom you can see free of charge, in most instances you would be expected to make some sort of contribution, often according to your means. There is some, but not very much, free individual psychotherapy available on the NHS (see p. 112), but only in certain areas. If you make arrangements to see a counsellor or psychotherapist privately check first on the fee (see p. 72).

There may be occasions when you need only a few sessions of therapy, either to sort out your feelings on a particular problem such as the illness of a close relative or fears of redundancy, for example, or to support you through a crisis. In such cases counselling, which concentrates on the here and now, is an appropriate form of help and can make all the difference to the way you cope. Most counsellors are flexible and will usually be prepared to see you just for a few sessions if you make it clear that that is what you want. Some of the voluntary counselling agencies also have particular skills in counselling certain types of problem such as bereavement and relationship difficulties, for example, and may be able to provide the help you need (see Chapter 18).

However, if you are considering counselling or psychotherapy over a longer period you might expect to have one or two exploratory sessions with the therapist concerned to see whether this seemed to be the right sort of help for you and, if so, whether you could work well together and what your aims should be. Your therapist needs to be someone you can respect and trust. If by any unfortunate chance you take an instant dislike to him or her or feel you are temperamentally unsuited, you are not going to get the most from therapy; it would then be quite reasonable for you to ask to see someone else.

Because therapy can be an up and down process, it often makes sense to make a commitment for a certain amount of time and then to review the situation with the therapist.

The introductory session with the therapist should dispel any lingering fears or misconceptions you have about the nature of individual therapy. Counsellors and psychotherapists are not there to interrogate you, to try to catch you out or to mystify you with fanciful and far-fetched interpretations of your behaviour, as people sometimes claim. Their role is to listen carefully and caringly to what you have to say, without making judgements about you, and to support you while you work through your problems at your own pace, offering suggestions from time to time to help you clarify your thoughts and feelings.

You should not expect your therapist to give you advice or tell you what to do. The aim of therapy is to help you gain a clearer idea of who you are and what you want from life so that you can make your own choices and devise your own strategies to cope with situations. Many people find that as therapy progresses they feel less boxed in by circumstances. As they change and gain in confidence, they begin to see situations in a new light or realize that different options are open to them.

Don't expect to learn much about your therapist at a personal level. Unlike friends, therapists will not share their own experiences or problems with you. The whole point of individual therapy is that it is an opportunity to focus on your needs and on you as an individual. The therapist will try to put him- or herself in your shoes in order to understand more completely your feelings and your situation, while at the same time remaining detached enough to support you while you find a way through. In fact, once you are used to it you may find it much easier to talk freely and openly to someone you do not know well and who is not judging you as a friend might do, especially as you are sure that everything you say will be treated in complete confidence.

The therapist's aim will be to establish a relationship with you in which you feel safe enough gradually to expose more of your real self and in which you can begin to look at your fears and anxieties as well as get in touch with and accept your real feelings. You may find it upsetting to talk about certain thoughts or experiences or express certain feelings for the first time but the therapist is there to support you and later you will probably feel a sense of relief. Fears are generally less threatening once they have been voiced and feelings that can be expressed are generally more manageable. Therapists are able to handle your distress because of their own training and professional support and because they are not emotionally involved with you in the same way as a friend or relative.

Of course, individual therapy might not necessarily be appropriate for you. You may not like the idea of a one-to-one approach and may feel more comfortable with group therapy (see p. 111); you may feel that firm advice and support are what you most need at this particular time; or that you prefer to find help in your own particular way, perhaps through a social or artistic activity, or through meditation or a sport, for example.

Group therapy

Like individual therapy, group therapy can be helpful for a wide range of mental health problems. You may find it particularly useful if you have difficulty in mixing easily with others and in forming relationships. It may not be advisable, however, if you feel highly insecure, perhaps due to a very deprived childhood. In that case individual therapy, which can focus solely on your needs, is probably a better way to build up your confidence.

A group, which may be led by one or two therapists, normally consists of between six and ten people of both sexes and with a range of difficulties. Some groups are known as closed groups. This means everyone starts group therapy at the same time and finishes together at the end of an agreed period. Other groups are known as open. This means they are continuous with new people joining as others leave.

If you start group therapy you are expected to regard it as a major commitment and not to miss a session unless you have very good reason. Group therapy is very much a sharing experience and you will have a responsibility to the other group members as well as to yourself. You will also be expected to treat anything discussed in the group as completely confidential.

In group therapy you will sit on chairs in a circle with the therapists, who will probably try to adopt a fairly unobtrusive role. They may help clarify the discussion or offer interpretations, for example, but the main aim will be to encourage group members themselves to share their difficulties and offer each other their own suggestions and insights. There may be periods of silence and if so you should not necessarily expect the therapist to intervene.

Group therapy consists, therefore, not just of working

through your own problems but also of helping others to work through theirs. Many people find that they learn a great deal by listening very carefully to others in a group setting, whether it is their own or someone else's problems that are being discussed. By working with others in this close way they also gain confidence about making relationships.

You will find that nearly everyone has the same worries and reservations before starting group therapy. It is quite normal to feel anxious at the thought of talking about yourself in front of strangers. But there is no need to disclose very much until you feel comfortable. Usually the realization that everyone is in the same boat gives people the confidence to start opening up.

Many people find that the experience of trying to look honestly at their difficulties in the company of others who are trying to do the same is a tremendous source of strength. They are also often reassured to discover that many of their fears and feelings, which they thought were abnormal, are in fact understood and shared by others. Participating in a group can also give people a sense of belonging and help overcome their feelings of isolation.

A group offers the opportunity, in a safe setting, to learn a great deal about ourselves at a social level, and how we come across to other people. Most people find it easier to accept criticism and suggestions that they might change within a group because a great deal of support is offered at the same time.

Psychotherapy and group therapy on the NHS

If your GP refers you to a psychiatrist who thinks you may benefit from either individual or group therapy, and this is available on the NHS in your area, then he or she may arrange for you to see a consultant psychotherapist. A consultant psychotherapist is a psychiatrist who has an additional recognized training in psychotherapy. You will be seen either by the consultant or by a psychotherapist in the team who may, or may not, be a doctor.

Questions in the interview are likely to be fairly open-ended to give you the opportunity to talk about your childhood and later life, your feelings and the way you experience your difficulties. If it seems that therapy might be helpful then one of the aims of the interview might be to decide whether individual or group therapy would be more appropriate, assuming that there is a choice.

If you are offered individual psychotherapy, it is likely to be once a week for fifty minutes. There may be a waiting list of between six months and two years. If there is no individual psychotherapy available or the waiting list is too long, you could ask to be referred privately if you can afford it.

If you are offered group psychotherapy it is likely to be once a week for between one and one and a half hours. Again, the waiting list may be between six months and two years. If there is no suitable group for you you could ask your psychotherapist about private groups. Some do exist in London and a few other centres.

CHAPTER 10

Behaviour-based Therapies

If you find yourself habitually responding to certain anxieties or situations in a way which in itself causes you distress, then behaviour therapy or therapy involving behaviour-based skills may be recommended. This approach can be helpful for many difficulties, including phobias, compulsive rituals and social skills problems, for example.

Behaviour therapy

People who know nothing about behaviour therapy often find the idea rather alarming. They may even worry that it might be associated with practices such as brainwashing. Quite the reverse is true in fact. Behaviour therapy is an extremely practical and common-sense approach in which your motivation and co-operation are essential; it is not something that can be done to you against your will.

Behaviour therapy focuses very much on the present and on the actual symptoms and reactions that are upsetting you. It looks closely at your behaviour in order to help you find an alternative way of responding that will cause you less distress.

In behaviour therapy you will work actively with your therapist, who may be a clinical psychologist, a nurse therapist or other suitably-trained professional worker, in order to try and identify your problem and find the best means of tackling it. This may be through one or more of a range of techniques, some of which are allied to some form of relaxation therapy, or through common-sense methods agreed by you and your therapist, or both. Talking to the therapist usually forms an important part of the treatment.

Behaviour therapy and psychotherapy should not be seen as two opposing methods, as is sometimes suggested; they are simply two different ways of approaching problems. Sometimes one method may be more suitable and sometimes the other and sometimes a mixture of the two. Most therapists practising behaviour therapy will also have counselling or psychotherapy skills, which they will use if appropriate.

The first session or two will be devoted to assessment to enable the therapist to decide whether behaviour therapy or some other approach might be the most helpful for you. These sessions are also an opportunity for you to find out whether behaviour therapy is a method you could work well with.

In these first meetings you are likely to be asked to describe your behaviour leading up to, during and following your distress in great factual detail. This may help you and the therapist to identify the strategies you are currently adopting to deal with the problem, its effects on you and those around you, and possible triggers for your difficulties. You may be asked to keep a diary in between sessions to help with this process and to pin-point factors that increase and decrease your anxiety, or you may be asked to monitor your anxiety regularly on a scale of one to ten throughout the day to see if there is a pattern to your reactions.

If at the end of the assessment you and the therapist agree that behaviour therapy might be helpful for you, you will then discuss what your aims will be. These are often quite precise, such as being able to do the shopping by yourself or travelling six stops by bus on your own. You would also expect to talk about the methods that might be used and the number of sessions likely to be involved.

Behaviour therapy is not a lengthy form of therapy. It is usually clear at a fairly early stage whether or not it is likely to be helpful. If it is, then you will probably achieve a satisfactory improvement with between ten and twenty sessions, or less. Moreover, the confidence thus gained is likely to spill over and benefit other areas of your life as well.

You are likely to see a therapist once a week at first for about an hour, with longer intervals between sessions as therapy progresses and you become more confident about managing your own treatment. You will often be given tasks to carry out at home and a friend or relative may be encouraged to help with these if they are willing. If relaxation forms part of the treatment you will be taught a suitable method (see Chapter 12) and asked to practise regularly at home until you are able to induce a state of relaxation quickly and easily, even in tense circumstances.

A few of the more common techniques you may come across in behaviour therapy are described here, and you should not be put off by their titles; there is nothing complicated about them. Incidentally, aversion therapy – an early technique that aimed to discourage unwanted behaviour by associating it with an unpleasant stimulus – is very rarely used nowadays.

Desensitization

One of the most widely used behaviour therapy techniques is known as desensitization or systematic desensitization. It is particularly helpful for certain phobias. First you are taught a relaxation method, and then asked to list the situations that make you anxious, starting with the least threatening and gradually building up to the one which terrifies you the most. If you have a cat phobia, for example, you might begin with 'looking at a picture of a cat' and finish with 'holding an actual cat'. Then while you are in a suitably relaxed state you will confront the first item on your list. Although you will experience anxiety, the relaxation technique and your therapist's support will help you to cope. You may need to repeat this stage a number of times. Once you are sure that you can cope with that object or situation without becoming too anxious you will move on to the next item, and so on, until you have overcome your fear. Some people find it helpful to work through the items in their imagination first before moving on to gradually confronting them in reality.

Exposure treatment

Another common method is known as exposure treatment or flooding. Here you are encouraged to confront whatever you find most frightening immediately and to remain in that situation for a considerable time – perhaps an hour – until your anxiety naturally subsides. This is a very effective method for many people and more effective if real situations are used rather than imaginary ones. For example, if you have a fear of shops you might go to a busy shop on several occasions and stay there, with your therapist close at hand to support you. Then, when you feel a little less frightened, you might try going with a friend and then finally on your own, until you can handle the situation without too much anxiety.

If, however, you feel more comfortable with a more gradual form of exposure, you and the therapist may decide on more limited targets each week. For example, if you are afraid of going out alone you might aim to get as far as your garden gate the first week, the pillar box the next week, the shops the third week and so on.

If you suffer from compulsions, you might be placed in

circumstances that normally give rise to your compulsive behaviour. You would be persuaded to refrain from carrying out your normal rituals for as long as possible while anxiety first mounts and then subsides and you realize that nothing dreadful occurs if the ritual is omitted. This process is repeated for gradually lengthening periods of time until you are able to dispense with the compulsive behaviour. You will require a great deal of support from your therapist and from friends and relatives during this period.

Operant conditioning

Another fairly widely used technique to encourage more desirable forms of behaviour, especially with children, is known as operant conditioning. This simply means that acceptable behaviour is rewarded by praise, by stars or by a system of tokens that can be exchanged for a treat, for example, and undesirable behaviour is simply ignored.

Cognitive therapy

Cognitions, in this context, mean thoughts, and cognitive therapy or cognitive behaviour therapy, as it is sometimes termed, is about learning to think and consequently to behave in a more positive way. It is a type of behaviour therapy that has been found to be helpful for certain types of depression and anxiety.

For example, if you constantly see yourself and others in a negative light, and have gloomy thoughts about your past and future, you are likely to interpret situations and what people say to you in a way that makes you feel even more anxious or depressed. If someone is rude to you in a shop, for instance, you might see this as further proof that you are unlikeable. You would not consider the possibility that the person was harassed or just bad mannered. Even if someone pays you a compliment, you will convince yourself that they cannot really mean it; and if someone is unable to meet you for lunch on one occasion, you will be certain that it is because they do not really like you, rather than accepting that something important has cropped up.

When you have to make a journey alone, you may tend to focus on the fact that there is no one to go with you, rather than on the opportunity to see a new place or meet new people. Similarly, if you have to tackle a situation that makes you highly anxious, you may continually tell yourself you cannot cope, which then becomes a self-fulfilling prophecy.

In cognitive therapy you would work with the therapist – usually a clinical psychologist or nurse therapist – to identify those negative thoughts and beliefs that seem to be reinforcing your depression or anxiety and to try to find more positive approaches. If you think cognitive therapy might be helpful for you, ask your GP or psychiatrist if it is available in your area.

Like ordinary behaviour therapy, cognitive therapy is a fairly quick method of treatment, often involving only about twelve one-hour sessions, as well as tasks to do at home. Sessions may be spaced at weekly intervals at first, and then more widely apart as your confidence improves.

The initial session or sessions for assessment are to enable you and the therapist to decide whether cognitive therapy might be helpful for you. If you continue, you might expect the therapist to use a number of methods to help you recognize the way you think and become more flexible and positive in the way you view yourself and others. You might be asked to keep a diary so that you can understand your own negative patterns of thought more clearly, and what their consequences are for you. It may also help you identify certain areas of your life that you find satisfying so that you can begin to build on these.

In cognitive therapy you should expect to have your ideas constantly challenged by the therapist, and learn to challenge them yourself. For example, the therapist may ask you to list all the arguments you can think of to back up your assertion that there is no point in going for a walk, and then challenge you on each of these, or you may be asked to provide arguments for and against your own view.

Quite often the therapist will ask you to test out a negative idea in practice, such as telephoning a friend whom you are sure does not want to speak to you. You should gradually become accustomed to replacing negative statements such as 'There is no way I can manage this' with more realistic, positive ones such as 'I know this will make me anxious but I'll take it step by step.' Your therapist may also use role play or relaxation methods to help you find better strategies to cope.

Social skills training

Most of us could do with some help in improving our social skills in order to interact more pleasantly and confidently with others. Perhaps we have an abrupt telephone manner, for example, have difficulty in making a complaint or are always overcome with shyness at a party, although one or two deficiencies will not usually prevent us from coping reasonably well in life. However, it is far harder to manage if for some reason we have missed out on learning a whole range of basic social skills as we were growing up, so that we have very little idea as to what behaviour others expect from us or how we should respond to them. This can lead to difficulties in forming relationships and getting on with people generally, which, in turn, may contribute to feelings of isolation and mental distress. People who have become so overwhelmed by a mental health problem that they have lost confidence in using the social skills they once had may find themselves very much in the same position.

In either of these cases your GP, psychiatrist or social worker may suggest that you join a social skills group at your local psychiatric hospital or unit, or in the community. The group will probably consist of about eight to ten people and one or two therapists, who may be occupational therapists, clinical psychologists or other professional workers in the mental health field. You are likely to meet regularly once a week for about an hour and a half and to be given tasks to practise at home with the help of friends and relatives.

The therapists may use a number of different techniques, such as copying – sometimes called modelling – and role play, to help you interact more closely with other people and tackle new situations. You will probably start by practising skills of communication, such as body language, including eye contact and facial expression; tone of voice; initiating conversation and responding appropriately. Later, you may move on to practising ways of handling situations you find difficult, such as asking for something in a shop, making a telephone inquiry or going for an interview, taking it in turns to play different roles and commenting on each other's performances. Sometimes a video is used to help you see more clearly what you are doing.

When you feel confident enough you will be asked to try out your skills in real situations and discuss them with the group the following week. The discussions will provide you with support and encouragement as you gradually acquire more skills and become more independent.

Assertiveness training

Being assertive should not be confused with being aggressive, overbearing or selfish. It simply means taking your own needs seriously because you value yourself as a person, and making this clear to others. If you are mentally distressed and have great difficulty in expressing your own wishes and needs, it might be suggested that you join an assertiveness group or that assertiveness training forms some part of your therapy.

In assertiveness training you will learn a number of skills through discussion, exercises and role play to enable you to express your needs and feelings more clearly, calmly and confidently. You might, for example, practise ways of making a request for yourself, of saying no in a difficult situation, of giving and receiving criticism or of giving and receiving compliments. You will also be encouraged to test your skills in actual situations.

Many people find assertiveness training useful as it helps them to come to terms with the idea that it is quite acceptable to disappoint others sometimes or to make mistakes. If they tend to set themselves rather too high standards, this can give them a new sense of freedom as well as confidence.

Many people who are not distressed enough to seek therapy but who nevertheless lack confidence in one or two areas may also benefit from assertiveness training. Assertiveness courses are often run by adult education departments of local authorities as well as by other organizations. You can find details at your local library.

Family therapy

When children or young adolescents show signs of being distressed, parents and other members of the family are usually closely involved. It makes sense, therefore, for therapists to talk to the whole family to try to uncover reasons for the distress, and to work out with them ways in which everyone can help. Family therapy is less commonly used with older adolescents, who usually prefer to see a therapist individually to preserve their privacy.

Family therapy is widely available on the NHS at child guidance clinics and hospital-based child psychiatric clinics. Your GP can refer you for family therapy or you can refer yourself to a child guidance clinic (see Chapter 5). You will only need to give brief details, which should include the nature of the problem as you see it – for example, bed wetting, school refusal or unmanageable behaviour – how long it has been going on for and, of course, your child's name, age and sex. If there has been a recent event that may have been upsetting to your child, such as a divorce, a death in the family, the arrival of a new baby or a move, it would be sensible to mention this too.

Some parents feel quite unnecessarily ashamed of seeking help in this way. They see it as a sign of failure. But quite the reverse is true. Recognizing that something is wrong and getting the appropriate help is an essential first step. Everyone finds bringing up children difficult at times, particularly where there are unexpected stresses and strains. Most parents will admit that there are occasions when they would welcome assistance if only to reassure them that they are doing all they can.

Family therapy can be thought of rather like a round table conference. Each member of the family views the problem in a rather different way, and each may be aware of an aspect that the others do not know of. It is not just that it is the most sensible and most economical use of the therapist's time to see the family together; members of the family themselves can benefit from seeing the problem from new angles and from having the opportunity to say what they feel, to discuss helpful suggestions and to correct each other's misunderstandings.

The first interview will probably be a family appointment

for both parents, unless you are a single parent family, the child concerned, brothers and sisters and any other close family members who wish to be involved. The therapist may be a child psychiatrist, a child psychotherapist, a psychologist, a social worker or family therapist. Sometimes two therapists may be present. The interview will probably last about an hour and you should regard it as an opportunity to discuss whatever is worrying you, however trivial it may seem.

Besides wanting to hear about how each of you sees the problem, the therapist will also be trying to find out how you behave as a family in order to suggest alternative approaches that make sense and feel right for you. After all, there is no one correct way to bring up children; all families operate differently and there are many different approaches that may be equally acceptable. Sometimes an additional therapist may observe your reactions to each other through a one-way screen in order to offer another viewpoint.

Family therapy does not ask you to delve into your deeper feelings or look back too much into the past. Instead, it helps you to examine very carefully what is happening now so that you can find new ways of coping. If a child is refusing to go to school, for example, each member of the family might be asked to give an account of their individual actions from getting up in the morning to the time when the confrontation takes place. Then, on the basis of their pooled information, the family might jointly decide to see if it is helpful for everyone to sit down to breakfast together to provide a calmer atmosphere, or whether it makes a difference if someone gets up a little earlier to give the child in question some extra attention. Sometimes small shifts in everyone's behaviour can make all the difference to a problem.

Quite often during family therapy it becomes apparent

that what the family has seen as the child's problem is simply his or her way of showing anxiety about stresses within the family that other members of the family may not have openly acknowledged. These stresses may be due to worries over employment, the birth of another child, the illness of a relative or tension between parents, for example. Once the family recognizes this and is able to talk about the real stresses more openly, it often lifts the burden from the child.

You may find that one session is enough to clarify the problem and enable you to handle it, or you may find that several sessions would be more helpful. Sometimes the therapist may recommend other means of help that might be appropriate, such as individual therapy for the child or marital therapy for the parents.

A gap of several weeks is normally left between family therapy sessions to enable the family to try out any ideas discussed with the therapist, as well as other ideas that may have occurred to them. Many families find that four or five sessions are enough to make a considerable difference. They can contact the therapist again even when the therapy has ended, if further difficulties arise.

Adult family therapy

Although family therapy is far more widely practised for children, it is also useful when older people are distressed and the family is so closely involved that it is hard to see what the problems actually are. Everyone needs support to stand back a little and see the situation more clearly. Your GP, psychiatrist or social worker may refer you for family therapy if it is available and appropriate to your particular situation.

CHAPTER 11

Hospital Care

You are now far less likely to spend time in hospital if you are diagnosed as suffering from a mental illness than you were ten or twenty years ago, and even if you are admitted, your stay will probably be a much shorter one. There are a number of reasons for these changes.

Firstly, more doctors and other health professionals recognize that it is less disturbing for people to remain in their own homes and receive treatment from their GPs or on an out-patient basis wherever this is possible. Secondly, the development of certain drugs since the late 1950s that help to control the symptoms of various forms of mental illness (see Chapter 8), as well as the availability of other forms of therapy, have meant that many people can lead more normal lives in the community while receiving treatment. Finally, the widely held view that community care can offer a better quality of life than long-stay hospital care has led to the gradual run-down of large, long-stay psychiatric hospitals, so that there are now fewer beds available.

Unfortunately, the provision of community care in England and Wales has not kept pace with the closure of beds and is extremely patchy, though there are some excellent schemes. In fact, the care you will be offered may depend more on where you live than the extent of your need. In many places alternative facilities to hospital care, such as various types of accommodation, day care and drop-in centres and sheltered workshops are just not available; nor are there sufficient numbers of social workers, community psychiatric nurses, occupational therapists or home helps to meet the demand.

Often, families are left to cope as best they can, or people simply slip through the net and struggle on their own. If you have a relative with a mental health problem and are living in an area where resources are scarce, you may have to work quite hard to get the help and support you need. Ask around and be persistent (see Chapter 18). There may be local or national voluntary organizations that can assist you or a local self-help or support group.

Scotland and Northern Ireland do not seem to be facing quite the same problems with community care, as they are reducing their hospital psychiatric beds much more gradually.

In-patient care

Although psychiatrists are less willing to admit people to hospital than some years ago, there are still good reasons why they may wish to do so. They may want to make a careful assessment before deciding on treatment and need to have you under observation. You may have a condition such as anorexia or suffer from an addiction and need constant support and monitoring. You may be feeling so distressed, or your behaviour may be so disturbed, that hospital care is the best alternative, or you may be admitted because there is no one to look after you or your family is no longer able to cope. You may also come into hospital, voluntarily or compulsorily (see Chapter 16), because it is feared you may be a danger to yourself or others.

The vast majority of psychiatric patients are voluntary patients. If you are a voluntary patient, it means you have talked the matter over with your doctor and agreed of your own free will to come into hospital. As a voluntary patient you have the right to refuse treatment or to discharge yourself, but it would always be sensible to discuss such decisions with the staff first. If you are a detained patient, the situation is rather different, but you still have certain rights (see Chapter 16).

You may be admitted to one of the larger, old-style psychiatric hospitals, many of which are now in the process of being run down, or to a psychiatric unit at your district general hospital. If you have never been in a psychiatric hospital or unit before it is likely that you or your relatives may be feeling rather apprehensive; it will therefore help to have as much information as possible.

Many hospitals issue information booklets giving details on visiting times, what to bring in with you, how to make a complaint and so on. You can also ring the nurse in charge of the ward and request any information you need. Patients normally wear day clothes in the daytime, but as lockers are usually quite small, you may want to check on what would be most useful to bring. Incidentally, doctors and nurses on many psychiatric wards now wear ordinary clothes, so don't be surprised not to see white coats or uniforms. Most people feel that it makes for a friendlier atmosphere.

Apart from the individual treatment you receive in hospital, which your psychiatrist will discuss with you, there is likely to be a weekly programme of activities in each ward that will form part of the overall treatment plan. It may include occupational therapy, art and music therapy, group therapy and ward discussions. You will be encouraged to participate if you feel well enough.

Relatives

If you are a relative you are likely to have quite mixed feelings when you leave someone in hospital. For example, although you may feel relieved that you no longer have the responsibility for a time, you may be rather ashamed of this reaction. You may feel guilty because you couldn't cope, or even angry with the patient for all the worry and upset you have gone through. Just remember that these feelings are quite normal, as you have probably been under a great deal of stress. Use this period to get your own strength back and accept that you may now need some support for yourself, either from family and friends or from your doctor.

There are often no restrictions on visiting in psychiatric wards, but do check first to make sure what the arrangements are, and that your visit does not clash with some organized activity. Try to visit as often as possible. It is the best way to help someone keep in touch with the outside world. You should try not to be put off if you are met with a hostile or apathetic response. It may be upsetting not to be greeted with open arms, perhaps after a long journey, but remember the person you are visiting is there because life has become difficult. Things won't miraculously change overnight. However, most people, when they recover, do say how important it was that those close to them kept on visiting, despite their behaviour at the time.

As the person improves, friends should be encouraged to visit too. They may be too afraid of intruding to suggest it, so it will help if you are quite open and matter of fact. If you are not embarrassed, then there is no reason why they should be.

Evenings and weekends can often seem to stretch interminably in hospital. When someone is well enough, it is often a good idea to go out for a walk or a meal. Quite often people are allowed home for a day or weekend to maintain the link with ordinary life or to prepare for leaving hospital.

If you are a close relative you will naturally want to be kept informed about treatment and progress although, of course, you will realize that certain details are confidential between the patient and psychiatrist. You can ask to see the psychiatrist or one of the other doctors in the team to talk about such matters, and ways in which you can be most helpful. However, don't be disappointed not to receive definite answers to questions such as how long treatment will take, or whether recovery will be complete. Individuals respond to treatment in different ways, and the extent of recovery may depend on a number of factors, some of which the doctor is unable to predict. He or she may prefer to be cautious rather than raise your expectations.

Nurses on the wards will generally make time to talk to both patients and relatives about any day-to-day practical problems and stresses; a hospital social worker is usually available as well to help sort out worries over matters such as benefits, housing or family problems, for example. It is often a good idea for either the patient or relative, or both, to see the hospital social worker before the patient is discharged to make sure there are satisfactory arrangements for accommodation, day-time activities and ongoing support, for instance.

Discharge

When you are discharged from hospital it will be to the care of your GP though you may still be under the psychiatrist's care for follow-up visits to the out-patients department or for other forms of therapy arranged by the psychiatrist.

It often helps if families are prepared for the period following a patient's discharge to be rather a tricky one. Decisions may have had to be taken in that person's absence and readjustments may have to be made by the whole family when he or she returns.

It is all too easy to assume that everything will be exactly as it was before the person was ill, forgetting that they may need a long time to recuperate and build up their confidence again. In some cases, of course, things will remain very different and everyone in the family will need to come to terms with this and adapt.

Although probably not as worrying as before the person went into hospital, this can be a stressful time. If you are a close relative, it may help if you can express any strong feelings you may have such as anger or exasperation to a trusted friend rather than bottling them up or exploding at the person concerned.

If the situation does become very strained, do ask for help from your GP; it is hard to bear all the load on your own.

Day hospitals

If your psychiatrist thinks you can manage at home or your family is able to look after you, then he or she may suggest you attend a day hospital rather than being admitted as an in-patient. The treatment and routine will be similar to that on the ward, but you will go home each day.

Complaints

If you or a relative wish to complain about your medical treatment or care, either as a hospital in-patient or out-patient, first talk it over with the staff concerned. You may find that there has been a misunderstanding, or you may be satisfied with an explanation and apology. However, if you are unable to sort it out and you wish to take it further, put your complaint in writing either to the hospital manager or administrator, or to the consultant in charge of your case, keeping a copy. Making a complaint can be very complicated so seek advice from your local Community Health Council in England and Wales (see Chapter 18), from the Mental Welfare Commission in Scotland (see Chapter 16), or from your local Health and Social Services Board in Northern Ireland (the address will be in your local telephone directory).

PART III:

SELF-HELP AND INFORMATION

Although certain forms of treatment can be crucial in dealing with mental health problems, what happens in everyday life is also vitally important. The support of friends and relatives, for example, is one of the main factors in helping people come to terms with their problems and cope.

These chapters look at various methods of self-help, as well as at mental health legislation, financial problems and mental health terms. Useful organizations are described and particular attention is paid to close friends and relatives who are shouldering most of the responsibility for care in the community, often with little outside help or guidance or, indeed, recognition for their efforts. It is important that carers get support for themselves and pay attention to their own needs; otherwise they are at risk of developing mental health problems themselves.

CHAPTER 12

Keeping Fit

Keeping fit may seem a very low priority when people are either mentally distressed themselves or highly anxious as carers, but in fact our minds and bodies interact so closely that any improvements to our physical condition are likely to have a beneficial effect on our mental state. Greater physical well-being may not in itself solve the problems or remove the worries, but it can alleviate some of the stress and help people to cope.

Of course, anyone with mental health problems who is feeling very low or agitated will not be able to envisage taking a brisk walk or planning a balanced meal. These are suggestions, therefore, for them to consider as they begin to get better, encouraged, where possible, by those close to them.

Those who are caring for someone with mental health problems can quickly become tense and exhausted themselves and feel quite overwhelmed by the situation. They need to take particular care of their own health if they are to continue to offer support as well as manage the other areas of their life satisfactorily. If they are fit and able to relax, they will have more energy to draw on and are more likely to be able to stand back and see things in perspective.

Diet

It is more important than ever to eat regular, well-balanced meals when you are stressed. Missing meals or having an inadequate diet can increase anxiety or depression, and reduce energy levels. Equally, overeating, for comfort's sake, can bring weight problems, which may in turn contribute to depression.

It is generally agreed that most people in this country have too much fat and sugar in their diet and too little fibre, and that this often results in considerable health problems. Cutting down on your intake of sugary and fatty foods and eating more fresh foods and foods containing fibre, such as wholegrain cereals, wholemeal bread, fresh fruit and vegetables, will help to improve your general health and feeling of well-being and also help you keep your weight down.

Many people, particularly very elderly people, are quite resistant to the idea of making even minor changes in their diet for the sake of their health. If you are caring for someone with these views who is mentally distressed, and you feel some changes are essential, then you will need to introduce them very gradually and tactfully.

There are two groups of people who appear to be particularly vulnerable to eating problems associated with mental health. The first group is elderly people who live alone and seem depressed. Relatives and others in contact with such people will need to keep an eye on their diet, as they may lose interest in food or forget to eat properly. Their diet then becomes deficient in certain nutrients, such as vitamins and minerals, which in turn leads to further health problems.

The other group is young people who seem over-concerned with their weight and with food generally and who may be at risk of developing an eating disorder as a result of their anxiety. Both anorexia, which involves self-starvation, and bulimia, which involves episodes of insatiable eating, frequently start after a period of dieting and are extremely difficult to handle once they become entrenched. If you suspect someone close to you is suffering from either of these disorders, seek advice immediately (see Chapter 5).

Tea and coffee

Many of us increase the number of cups of tea or coffee we drink when we are stressed or anxious without realizing that these drinks may in fact be contributing to our anxiety. Tea and coffee contain substantial amounts of the drug caffeine, which is also present in cola drinks, cocoa, chocolate and some over-the-counter remedies.

Caffeine acts as a stimulant and a few cups of tea or coffee a day probably do little harm to most people. However, taken in larger quantities caffeine can result in unpleasant side-effects, such as headaches, irritability, restlessness, dizziness, hand tremors, palpitations and anxiety, although anyone suffering these symptoms may not recognize that caffeine is the cause, and may increase their intake in order to keep going.

How many caffeine-containing drinks you can consume each day without adverse effects depends on a variety of factors, including the size of the cup, the strength of the brew and your own metabolism. As a very rough guide a large, strong cup of coffee will contain approximately twice as much caffeine as a large, strong cup of tea. If your consumption is fairly high or you are noticing unpleasant side-effects, you would be wise to cut down. You might try substituting other drinks, such as fruit juice, herb teas or even water.

Drugs

When your doctor prescribes a drug for you it is important to ask not just about its likely benefits to your health, but also about any possible side-effects, since all drugs have some side-effects. If you are worried by certain side-effects when you are taking the drug, you should discuss this with your doctor as soon as possible.

The situation with illegal drugs is rather different. People start using such drugs, not for health reasons, but for enjoyment, or as a temporary escape from stress or anxiety. However, they run the risk, with certain drugs, that they will become dependent, and endanger both their physical health and mental stability, as well as disrupting their work and family life. If you are worried because you are taking such drugs, or because someone close to you is using them, seek advice from your GP or from a helpful organization (see Chapter 18).

Of course, dependency, and its allied physical and mental health problems, does not occur only with illicit drugs. Many people have become unwittingly dependent on minor tranquillizers, for example, and may need a great deal of support should they wish to come off (see Chapter 8).

Alcohol

Because alcohol is so widely available and so socially acceptable it is easy to forget what a powerful drug it is. It acts as a sedative, lessening some of the restraints that normally govern our behaviour. Even small amounts can affect our judgement and concentration and, therefore, skills such as driving and operating a machine.

Drinking in moderation and at sensible times in a social setting is a pleasant and enjoyable means of relaxation for

many people. But they may need to look carefully at their
drinking habits, or seek help to do so, if they are beginning
to increase their drinking, finding they can't relax without a
drink, needing a drink earlier in the day or drinking frequently when alone.

What constitutes a reasonable level of alcohol for each
person depends on a variety of factors, including their
individual metabolism, their state of health and when the
alcohol is consumed. However, a figure that is commonly
recommended as a guide is a maximum of twenty-one units
for men and fourteen units for women, spread over a week.
A unit equals half a pint of beer, a single whisky or a glass
of white wine, according to pub measures. Some of the
extra-strong beers and lagers can be as much as three times
as strong as ordinary beer, and a half pint of one of these
may equal three units.

Unfortunately, many people drift into drinking more heavily when they are under stress or in an attempt to escape
from anxiety or depression. However, regular heavy drinking not only endangers health and puts people at risk of
becoming dependent on alcohol, but it also generates its
own mental health problems, often increasing depression
and anxiety and leaving people in a less fit state to cope. If
you find you are drinking too heavily, or using alcohol as a
crutch for your problems, it would be sensible to go to your
GP or to contact a helpful organization (see Chapter 18).

If you are taking medication for your mental health problems, you may not be able to drink any alcohol. Check with
your doctor.

Smoking

Even if you are a smoker you are no doubt well aware of the
health hazards associated with smoking. However, you also

need to realize that when you are under stress there is a temptation to increase the amount you smoke, thus increasing the dangers to your health and undermining your general fitness even further, without helping to solve your underlying problems.

Rather than smoking more heavily, try to find an alternative means of coping with your tension, such as taking a short walk, talking to a friend or doing a relaxation exercise.

You may wish to give up smoking altogether. If so, you should try to pick a period when you are less stressed and make sure you have plenty of support. Ask your GP for advice.

Exercise

Exercise is important not only for your physical health. It can also have a direct affect on your mood. Many people report that they feel less anxious or depressed after taking exercise, and as people become more fit they often become more confident and positive as well. Exercise is also a good way to relieve the tensions that accumulate during the day, whether you are caring for someone with mental stress or simply have a stressful occupation.

Exercise needs to be regular – that is at least two or three times a week – in order to be beneficial. It is important, therefore, to choose an activity you enjoy; otherwise it becomes a chore rather than a pleasure and you are less likely to continue with it.

If it is a new form of exercise for you, or if you are physically unfit you should build up gradually or you may damage yourself physically. If you are at all worried about a particular form of exercise because of a physical disability or illness, then consult your doctor first.

Regular exercise will increase the amount of energy the

body has available, but this does not mean that everyone should be encouraged to embark on strenuous activity. If you are feeling very low or exhausted, short gentle walks in the fresh air to get you moving and provide a change of scene will be more appropriate.

It is easy to feel very trapped when you are experiencing mental distress or caring for someone who is. Taking exercise can be a way of starting to take decisions for yourself and of beginning to exert some control over your own life.

Sleep

People vary in the amount of sleep they require, both as individuals and at different periods of their life. What is important is that each person should get enough for their own needs and wake refreshed. Unfortunately, many people with mental health problems also find they have sleeping difficulties just at the time when they most need the recuperative powers of sleep. Lack of sleep or broken, restless sleep means they wake exhausted or tense, feeling even less able to cope with daily life than before.

A common pattern for people with depression, for example, is to wake very early in the morning when spirits are at their lowest ebb and be unable to get back to sleep. With anxiety the difficulty is often in falling asleep initially; the mind races and the problems of the day magnify.

Obviously it is important to discuss any mental health problem with your GP and to mention your sleeping difficulties. But you should not expect a prescription for sleeping pills, except possibly for a very limited period (see Chapter 8). However, there are some measures you can take to help yourself, though you will need to find out through experience which are the most appropriate for you.

It is important to feel relaxed before you go to bed. Anyone will have difficulty in sleeping if their mind is over-active. It is often helpful, therefore, if you can switch off from your problems and spend the latter part of the evening in a not too demanding way. Avoiding eating a heavy meal or drinking tea, coffee or alcohol in the evening can also often help. Exercise during the day will enable you to feel physically tired and a walk before bed may make sleep easier. Some people find a hot bath in the evening helps them to relax; others may prefer listening to music, reading quietly or even sipping a warm, milky drink. Elderly people tend to need less sleep; they may find that going to bed a little later is helpful.

If you find that you are still tense when you are lying in bed, try not to worry about getting to sleep. You might try doing a relaxation exercise to calm you down. Even if you are unable to sleep, the fact that you are relaxed is beneficial.

Relaxation

Being able to relax is crucial for our physical and mental well being, particularly when we are stressed. Relaxation enables the body to recuperate and the mind to refresh itself, but it is precisely during those periods when we are emotionally tense and anxious that we have the most difficulty in relaxing. Tension builds up and we are likely to become even more irritable, angry or depressed with no outlet for our feelings.

One way of resolving this difficulty is through relaxation exercises. They will help you relax your body completely, and, in the process, your mind will also become calmer. Though underlying problems remain, you will probably feel better equipped to deal with them.

All relaxation exercises combine learning to breathe more

fully using the diaphragm and a method of muscular relaxation. One method involves tensing and relaxing the main muscles in turn, starting with the feet and moving upwards through the body to the head. This helps people recognize what a muscle feels like when it is tense and when it is fully relaxed. Another method involves concentrating on each part of the body in turn and feeling it become warm and heavy. Visualization is often used as an aid to relaxation. Conjuring up an image such as a flower or calm sea, or a happy peaceful event in the past, often helps people to relax more fully.

Once you have learned the relaxation technique, you will need to practise it regularly at home. When you have become accustomed to relaxing in this way, you should find that it becomes easier to relax at other times, even in stressful situations.

You can ask your GP or inquire at your local library about relaxation classes or tapes. Once you have discovered the benefits of relaxation, you may want to try other methods of deep relaxation, such as yoga or meditation. Again, you can inquire about classes at your local library.

CHAPTER 13

Helping Each Other

As hospital beds close and 'care in the community' becomes more widespread, each of us has even more responsibility to see in what ways we can make life more pleasant for people with mental health problems, and for those who are caring for them, so that they do indeed feel part of the community. Such efforts are particularly important because facilities in the community are so often inadequate.

Unfortunately, however, instead of helping, we often make life more difficult for people with mental health problems because of our own lack of understanding, embarrassment or prejudice. Moreover, very few of us make enough positive efforts to overcome the considerable and quite irrational stigma that still attaches to mental illness and causes so much unnecessary additional suffering. Stigma means a mark of shame or discredit, and all too often we find it easier to dismiss people with mental health problems as if they were in some way to blame for them, rather than trying to comprehend the true nature of their distress.

One result of these attitudes is that those suffering from mental illness and those close to them are likely to see it as something to be ashamed of and to be hidden from the world. Families will then tend to turn inwards and become more isolated, rather than looking outwards for support and leading a more normal life. They may view themselves as being in some way strange, not realizing just how wide-spread mental health problems are.

Self-help and support groups

One way of overcoming the feeling of stigma and sense of isolation is to join a self-help or support group, which can form a bridge between the home and the outside world (see Chapter 18). The rapid growth of such groups both for people with mental health problems and for their relatives or carers has been one of the most positive developments in the mental health field in recent years.

The understanding and support of those who have faced the same problems and experienced the same feelings is often one of the most important factors in enabling people to come to terms and to cope. Such groups can help overcome the loneliness and hopelessness that many people feel whether they are distressed themselves or closely involved with someone who is. They can also give people the opportunity to make sense of their own experiences through helping others.

Group members support each other through listening, through encouragement and through suggesting various alternative strategies. Humour is an important safety valve when you are under stress and such meetings often enable you to see the funny side of situations. Being accepted for exactly who you are can also be a great source of strength; it can give you the confidence to talk more openly about your difficulties and experiences, either to friends or more widely afield, so that public understanding of mental health problems is gradually improved.

Friends and neighbours

If you are a friend or neighbour of someone who is mentally distressed, you may wish to offer help but feel uncertain as to what might be appropriate. Sadly, many people end up doing nothing out of embarrassment, leaving those with mental health problems feeling even more isolated and rejected.

The first thing to remember is that everyone feels helpless and inadequate in the face of mental distress, and that your role is simply to offer support, not find a solution. There is no need to undertake anything large or to overcommit yourself; just sitting listening to someone for an hour from time to time or making a phone call once a week can often make an enormous difference. The person concerned may seem unresponsive, but the message you are giving them is that they do matter, and that is extremely important. Many people, when they recover, say that gestures such as these were a lifeline.

It is also important to remember that many mental health problems take a long time to resolve themselves, even with treatment. If you are offering support, you should not feel discouraged because you cannot see any improvements or because the person seems to have slipped back, rather than progressed. Your help is still of value.

Listening

When someone is distressed, they usually find it a great relief to talk about their feelings. You can help them feel safe enough to do so by listening with your full attention and without making any judgements. Someone in this sort of state is not really looking for advice or logical answers to their problems. What they are really seeking is reassurance at a deeper level. Simply showing you understand what they feel by your warmth and concern is enough. Advising them to snap out of it, on the other hand, or refusing to accept that they really feel so bad may make you feel better but will almost certainly make them feel worse.

This is not really the time to share your own experiences as you might normally do with a friend. The person concerned will be so absorbed by their own feelings that they will not want to focus on anything else. You will also need to avoid the temptation to indulge in any amateur psychology. What is wanted at this stage is your total support, not an analysis of what might or might not have occurred.

You may feel as if you are doing very little by simply listening but giving someone your time and attention like this is often the most helpful thing you can do.

Touching

Sometimes people may not feel like talking or you may not know what to say. Then sitting just holding their hands may be more appropriate. Most people who are distressed do, in fact, crave some sign of physical warmth, though they often lack the confidence to make an affectionate gesture themselves. Of course, you need to use your judgement, but often giving a hug or putting your arm round someone is immensely comforting. A warm human contact confirms they are valued and approved of for themselves.

Practical help

You may prefer to offer assistance at a practical level. Collecting the children from school, doing some shopping or even cooking an occasional meal, for example, can all be ways of alleviating someone's stress. Keeping someone company to relieve a relative who feels tied is another very worthwhile form of help.

However, it is also important to exercise tact when offering practical help. Find out, if possible, what the person concerned would really like you to do so that it does not appear as though you are trying to take over. You may feel that cleaning the house would be the most useful contribution you could make. In some cases you might be right but in others it might be counter-productive; your very efficiency might make the person you are trying to help feel even more inadequate. Just helping with the washing up might then be more appropriate.

When people are distressed they often feel quite overwhelmed and unable to make decisions about what needs doing first. But if you listen carefully you may find that they are particularly bothered by some small task they have been unable to tackle, such as filling in a form or making a phone call. Helping them with this can often relieve a great deal of anxiety.

Mental health problems cause many people to function far more slowly. They may take several hours to complete a task that previously took them less than a quarter of the time. It is important not to impose your own expectations of what they might achieve. Do not force someone into an activity but if you can encourage them to work with you on a small task at their own rate it may benefit their self-esteem. You are then giving them company and support as well as practical help.

CHAPTER 14

Stresses for Friends and Relatives

If you are supporting someone with a mental health problem, then you are likely to be under considerable stress as well. It is important to recognize that this is a worrying time and to take particular care of yourself, both for your own sake and so that you can continue to offer support. It is crucial to marshall all the help you can rather than struggling to manage on your own. Try to bring in other members of the family or close friends to share some of the responsibility and make full use of whatever services are available.

Having someone you can talk to about your own anxieties and feelings can make all the difference whether it is your doctor, an understanding friend or relative, or a member of a self-help or support group. It can help you stay in touch with your own strengths and give you the confidence to cope.

Finding out all you can about the mental health problem in question can often be helpful in giving you some idea of what you might expect, though it is important to remember that each person will react in their own way. Many voluntary and self-help organizations issue useful information sheets and booklists (see Chapter 18).

Getting help

One of the first problems you are likely to face is trying to decide whether or not someone needs outside help. You will, of course, need to trust your own judgement and what you already know about the person. Generally speaking, you should try to persuade someone to see their GP if they seem very distressed or extremely withdrawn over a number of days or if their behaviour has altered without good reason so they are no longer coping with work or with daily activities or relationships.

If they are unwilling to visit the doctor, it might make sense for you to seek help yourself, either from an appropriate professional worker (see Chapter 7) or from a relevant organization (see Chapter 18), in order to find out the best way to handle the situation.

Sometimes you may persuade someone who is distressed to go for help, only to find that none is forthcoming. You may then need to be persistent on their behalf, if that is appropriate. You should not be put off by people who label you as 'over-anxious'. It is quite normal to be very anxious if someone close to you is exceedingly upset or behaving in a strange way. It is also sensible to ask for help at an early stage, when problems are easier to handle, rather than waiting for a crisis to erupt.

It is usual to experience shock or pain when someone close to you is diagnosed as having a mental health problem. However, this can often be followed by a feeling of relief because it helps to make sense of much otherwise inexplicable behaviour. Once the problem has been identified, you can start to think more clearly about the best ways to offer support and to handle the situation.

Blame

Relatives frequently blame themselves or feel guilty if someone close to them is mentally distressed. You may find that you are spending a lot of time going over the past, searching for an explanation in something you did or failed to do. Rather than worrying about possibly imaginary inadequacies, it makes more sense to build on the strengths of the relationship as it is now, and to look for new strategies to help you cope.

Unfortunately, relatives are also sometimes quite unfairly blamed for mental health problems either by the person suffering or even, occasionally, by mental health professionals. This is despite the fact that we know very little about the causes of most mental health problems.

Coming to terms

If mental health problems last for any length of time, there are certain aspects you will need to come to terms with. One is that progress, when it occurs, is often slow and uneven. Delight at a step forward is often dashed as the person slips back yet again. Rather than switching continually between over-optimism and despondency, most people eventually learn to adjust their expectations and take each day as it comes.

Even more difficult to handle is the fact that certain mental health problems can cause people to behave in unpredictable ways. No sooner have you adapted to one situation than a totally unexpected problem rears its head. It is important to accept that this is a source of considerable strain and to have as wide a network of support as possible to fall back on.

Everyone needs a break from caring, particularly when the sufferer has serious mental health problems. You could ask social services and local voluntary organizations (see Chapter 18) if they can provide information about day centres, holiday arrangements, clubs and respite care.

It is always painful to witness distress in someone close to you and be unable to help. If that distress is long-lasting and is also accompanied by changes in personality or capability, then you may need to work through feelings of grief and loss, rather as in a bereavement, before you can really accept the person as they are.

Detachment

It is essential to try to preserve a certain degree of detachment when someone is mentally distressed, however concerned you are. If you identify too closely with the difficulties and let yourself be drawn in, then you are likely to lose confidence too. There is a difference between saying to someone 'I understand that you see the world in this way' and trying to see it that way yourself. You will be much more help if your feet remain firmly planted on the ground.

You will also need to stand back a little in order to make yourself less vulnerable and avoid being hurt. People who are distressed are usually so weighed down by their own problems that they have no energy left to consider anyone else's needs. They may, as a result, reject your gestures of affection or appear quite uncaring or unresponsive; or they may criticize you remorselessly or display anger or hostility because you are the person on whom it is easiest to vent their feelings.

It is important to distinguish these sorts of behaviour from everyday ups and downs, and to realize that they are simply part of the mental distress. Although it is sometimes difficult, you should try not to take them personally. Your support and encouragement are still needed, but you, in turn, will need support and affection from other members of your family or friends; otherwise you will quickly become emotionally exhausted.

Independence

It is always hard to maintain just the right balance between offering help and encouraging independence when someone has mental health problems. The temptation is to take over completely, either because the person concerned wants you to do so or because it is quicker and easier. But, except in cases where people are extremely low or acutely distressed, this is not really helpful in the long run. Some measure of independence is crucial in order for people to regain confidence and find a way to cope with life on their own terms. You need to find a way of doing just enough to enable them to manage while still allowing them to do whatever they can for themselves, however long it takes.

Of course, if you have needed to be particularly vigilant at some stage of caring or have been put in the position of making all the decisions, it is even more difficult to step back, particularly if the worry is still at the back of your mind. However, if you can withdraw gradually as they begin to improve and spend more time on your own interests, while still offering support, it is likely to be better for everyone.

Coping strategies

Each person responds to a mental health problem in their own way and each relationship is unique, so there are no rules that you can follow in offering support. Of course, it is sensible to listen to advice from mental health professionals and to suggestions from people who have experience of similar problems, in self-help or support groups, for example. However, in the end you will have to rely on your own intuition and judgement and the fact that you know the person best.

You should not worry if you sometimes get things wrong; you will only be able to find what works by a process of trial and error. For example, if you can persuade someone who has been reluctant to leave the house to do some shopping and they appear to manage without great difficulty, then that is obviously something worth trying to repeat. If, however, they seem very flustered or distressed as a result, then it may be best left for a while.

Some people respond well to having their day structured and from encouragement to complete small tasks. For others this is too much pressure and they prefer not to have to think ahead. Most people with problems manage far better in a calm atmosphere. Their minds are in turmoil enough without having to cope with external tensions. Though you may need to control your own emotional responses and exercise a great deal more patience and tolerance than usual, this does not mean that you should not state your limits firmly and make it quite clear that you cannot put up with certain sorts of behaviour.

Perhaps the most useful adjustment that you yourself can make is in lowering your expectations, at least for the time being. Once you are able to abandon your set ideas of what progress ought to be achieved, you will reduce your level of anxiety and be able to respond more realistically to the person's actual needs. Moreover, you may find yourself experiencing unexpected pleasure at even very small steps forward.

Feelings

You should not be surprised if you experience strong feelings of anger, resentment or irritation, particularly if a mental health problem has lasted for a considerable time. After all, your life has been substantially affected and you are probably having to do a great deal more at a practical level as well as offering emotional support, often with little appreciation being shown. Sometimes the most trivial incident, such as not getting help in laying the table, may seem the last straw.

Although it is usually counter-productive to show your anger or irritation to the person concerned, since it is likely to upset them further and make it harder for them to cope, you should not bottle up your emotions. Expressing your feelings to someone you trust and who understands what you are going through can help to make them more manageable. Finding an outlet for day-to-day tensions, such as physical exercise, can also be helpful.

You need to be aware that it is stressful to assume the coping, caring role in a relationship, without any respite or opportunity to be childish, moody or unreasonable yourself, should you wish. Indeed, you may become so absorbed in trying to find the best way of handling someone else's problems that you forget that you have needs and problems of your own. Moreover, having to tread carefully all the time to avoid causing any upset means that it is easy to lose any sense of spontaneity. This is why, as someone begins to recover, you may find it difficult at first to adapt and respond more naturally. In addition, you may find that your own feelings, which you have kept in check during the crisis, bubble to the surface quite strongly once the pressure is eased, and that you need some extra support for yourself.

Time to yourself

One way of trying to stay in touch with your own needs and preserving some sense of spontaneity is to make sure you have some time to yourself each day, however brief, to recharge your batteries. This should be spent in doing exactly what you want, whether it is simply taking a leisurely bath, pursuing a hobby or sitting quietly with a cup of tea.

People sometimes feel guilty about having time to themselves when there are so many demands on them and when someone else's needs seem greater than their own, but it is important for relatives, or anyone else in a caring role, to realize that they can only do so much. If you are giving out all the time, you will not only become exhausted, you will also lose a sense of your own worth, and this in turn can lead to depression, anxiety and other problems. Making time for yourself is a means of safeguarding your emotional strength and retaining your self-esteem.

CHAPTER 15

Financial Worries

Worries can escalate, particularly financial worries, when you or a close relative has mental health problems. Good advice at an early stage may relieve some of your anxieties whether concerning debts, rescheduling a mortgage or simply managing on less income. If you are not sure who to turn to, then a good source of free and independent advice is your local Citizens Advice Bureau (CAB).

Bureau workers have wide experience in dealing with financial as well as other problems, and anything you say will, of course, be treated in complete confidence. They are also used to giving information and explanations in terms that can easily be understood. This is important, as the last thing you will feel like is struggling to cope with difficult jargon.

The CAB staff may be able to help you sort out the problem themselves, or they may refer you to other professionals or organizations that can give you the advice or help you need. About a third of CABs have an accountant on tap for special sessions, and about half have a solicitor available at certain times to give free advice. You can simply walk into a CAB and ask for advice; but check the opening hours first as they do vary.

Local neighbourhood advice centres can also offer advice on financial and other problems, or point you in the right direction; some local authorities also run advice centres.

Benefits

If you are suffering from a form of mental illness that precludes you from working, you are likely to qualify for a variety of benefits depending on your circumstances. You may also qualify for some benefits if you are working, but have a low income.

It will save time if before making inquiries about benefits you sit down and work out how much money you already have coming in each week, and what your outgoings are. These would include, for example, mortgage or rent, rates, food, heating, clothes and so on.

To find out which social security or other benefits you may be eligible for, ask at your local CAB, or social security office, or ring the DSS (Department of Social Security) Freeline. The Freeline service, which is, of course, free to callers, offers advice and information on benefits over the telephone, and is particularly useful if you are too busy to call round at an office or if you prefer the anonymity of a telephone call. (For telephone numbers see p. 188–9).

When you have decided which benefits to apply for you will need to fill in the appropriate forms. CABs and post offices will carry some forms, and forms for all social security benefits are available at your local social security office. Social security offices are listed in the telephone book under Health and Social Security or Social Security. If you can't get to the office you can telephone and ask for the appropriate forms to be sent to you.

Filling in forms to claim benefits can be quite complicated, so do not hesitate to ask for advice if you need it. Someone at the local social security office should be available to help, but you may have to wait quite a while if they are busy, so the local CAB may be the best place to go. If your claim is unsuccessful, but you believe that you have a good case, the CAB can advise you on how to appeal.

For certain benefits you may need a letter from your doctor about your mental health problem, and for some you may need to be examined by a doctor appointed by the DSS. In that case you will be told what to do by your local social security office.

Unfortunately, you may sometimes encounter hostility when claiming benefits from people who know little about mental health problems. Don't be put off: remember you have a right to your benefits.

Carers, too, may qualify for an allowance. If you are spending a significant amount of time caring for someone with a serious mental illness on an informal and unpaid basis, you may possibly be eligible for a benefit. Again, check with your local CAB, your local social security office or the DSS Freeline.

Hospital

Always let your social security office know if you or a close relative are going into hospital if benefits are being claimed; also let them know the date of discharge once you know it yourself.

If you are in hospital for some time your benefits may be reduced or withdrawn, as some of your needs are being met by the hospital. But if you go home, even for a day or so, let the local social security office know, as you may be entitled to the full rate of benefit for however short a period.

The hospital social worker should be able to help you sort out any general problems to do with benefits, or at least point you in the right direction.

Appointeeship

Sometimes a person who is receiving benefits is considered to be incapable of managing their own affairs. In that case the DSS can appoint someone to administer these benefits in the claimant's interest. Where possible, it is preferable that the person appointed should be a close relative, but it might also be a friend or neighbour or a caring professional.

If you feel it would be helpful for you to be appointed by the DSS on a particular person's behalf the first step is to contact your local DSS office. A visiting officer will then call to see both you and the person receiving the benefits to make sure that everything is in order. You may be asked to produce medical or other evidence that the person concerned is incapable of managing their affairs.

This system operates throughout the UK. The person appointed may resign, or the order may be revoked and someone else appointed if it is thought that things are not being managed in the best way for the person concerned.

Court of Protection

A DSS appointee can manage only income derived from benefits. When someone who is considered mentally incapable has income from other sources, or property or investments that require attention, then other means have to be found. One possible method is the Court of Protection, which may be the best solution for some people although it is not cheap.

A receiver – that is, someone responsible for handling the financial affairs on behalf of the person who has become mentally incapable – is appointed by the Court. The receiver is then accountable to the Court for the way decisions are taken and the way money is spent, which provides a safeguard for all those concerned.

Usually a close relative acts as the receiver, but it could be a suitable friend or neighbour, the local authority, a solicitor, accountant or bank manager. When no one can be found to act, the Court can order the Public Trustee to act as the receiver. The largest group of people coming under the Court of Protection are the elderly.

You can apply to the Court of Protection to become a receiver if the person who has become incapable either lives or has property in England or Wales, or both. To make initial inquiries, simply telephone, write or call in person (the address is on p. 207). For Northern Ireland you should contact the Office of Care and Protection (the address is on p. 207). Scotland has no Court of Protection, but the Accountant of Court fulfils much the same role. For advice on how to proceed in Scotland, consult a solicitor.

Enduring Power of Attorney

A person can come under the Court of Protection only when they have been judged mentally incapable of managing their money and financial affairs. However, the legislation, known as the Enduring Power of Attorney (which came into force in 1986), enables people who are now competent to plan ahead for the possibility that they may become mentally incapable. They can give an Enduring Power of Attorney to someone they would trust to manage their affairs if this should happen. This is done on a special form, and independent legal advice should always be sought.

Unlike an ordinary power of attorney, which becomes invalid if the person giving the power becomes mentally incapable, the Enduring Power of Attorney retains its validity. When the person who has been made the attorney believes that the person concerned is becoming mentally incapable, he or she notifies that person and certain closest relatives that they intend to register that power with the Court of Protection. This gives time for any objections to be lodged.

Once registration has taken place, the attorney must act in accordance with the terms laid down by the person who gave the power. Most of the time this will be without supervision, but in the last resort anyone who objects to the way the attorney is acting can approach the Court of Protection, who may then consider whether that person should remain as attorney.

Making a will

A will is valid only if the person making it is of sound mind, memory and understanding. However, this does not necessarily preclude people who are suffering from some form of mental illness from making a valid will, but it must be clear that they are able to appreciate what a will is, and what it does. They must also understand in general terms what it is they have to leave and who they should consider leaving it to, even if they decide subsequently not to do so.

If there is likely to be any doubt about the capacity of an individual to make a will, the solicitor should ensure that attached to the will is a report from a doctor – preferably a consultant psychiatrist – stating that the person making the will has the capacity to do so at the time of making it.

When a person does not have the capacity to make a will, the only way one can be made on their behalf is through the Court of Protection. To find out about this you can telephone, write or call in (see p. 207).

CHAPTER 16

Detained Patients and the Law

Many people worry that a visit to a psychiatrist means that they may be whisked into hospital against their will. But only a minority of people seen by a psychiatrist are admitted to hospital as in-patients, and of these, the vast majority – between 90 and 95 per cent – enter on a voluntary basis.

These voluntary patients are also known as informal patients, and they have the same rights as patients who are being treated in hospital for physical illness. For example, they can refuse treatment if they wish and they can discharge themselves, though it is usually advisable to discuss this with staff first and to make appropriate arrangements.

England and Wales

The Mental Health Act 1983 was an important step forward in mental health reform. Most of the legislation embodied in this Act refers to formal patients, that small group of people who are compulsorily detained in hospital. The Act outlines the grounds on which people can be detained, the various ways in which this can be carried out, the safeguards for detained patients and their rights of appeal.

Detained patients are not free to leave hospital when they choose and are subject to special rules regarding treatment and their right to refuse it (see Chapter 8). The hospital should provide oral and written information for detained patients on their main rights when they are admitted.

If you or a relative are compulsorily detained in hospital, you will not want to cope with additional anxieties because you do not understand the legal situation or because you are puzzled by the terms you hear used. If you are unable to get satisfactory explanations from hospital staff, the local Citizens Advice Bureau or MIND's Legal and Welfare Rights Department will be able to help you (see Chapter 18).

Scotland

In Scotland the legislation equivalent to the Mental Health Act 1983 is the Mental Health (Scotland) Act 1984. Scotland, of course, has a different legal system, so though the broad intention of the Act is the same, it differs in detail. For further information contact the Mental Welfare Commission (address on p. 207).

There is no system of Mental Health Review Tribunals in Scotland. Patients or relatives wishing to appeal against compulsory detention to an independent body can appeal either to a Sheriff or to the Mental Welfare Commission (see p. 174).

Northern Ireland

Although Northern Ireland has basically the same legal system as England and Wales there are often minor differences of legislation. Since 1972 almost all legislation has been in the form of Orders in Council.

The Mental Health (Northern Ireland) Order 1986 covers similar ground to the Mental Health Act 1983, but differs in certain details. For example, nearly all compulsorily detained patients are first admitted to hospital for up to

seven days assessment, renewable for a further seven days.
If a patient is then discharged without treatment that period
can be regarded as if it had never happened for the purpose
of a job interview, for instance, though it would have to be
declared in a court of law if requested. For further information contact the Northern Ireland Association for Mental
Health (address on p. 201).

Mental Health Act 1983 (England and Wales

Steps leading to compulsory detention

When a person is compulsorily detained or compulsory
detention is being considered various people may have a
role to play. These include the GP, preferably the patient's
own, a psychiatrist, an Approved Social Worker (ASW) (a
qualified social worker who has been trained and approved
by the local authority to deal with mental health problems)
and the patient's 'nearest' relative. In Scotland the equivalent of an Approved Social Worker is a Mental Health Officer
(MHO).

Who the 'nearest' relative is, is not always clear. The
Mental Health Act 1983 ranks relatives in a certain order of
closeness to the patient, but sometimes the person who lives
with or cares for the patient will take precedence and
become the nearest relative for the purpose of the Act only,
even if they are not related. Your social services department
should be able to advise you on this.

Applications for compulsory admission to hospital are
made by the nearest relative or an Approved Social Worker
on forms issued by the Department of Health. Approved
Social Workers normally keep a supply of forms and, in the
vast majority of cases, make the applications. The application must be supported by recommendations in writing from
two doctors who have examined the patient; one of these

doctors must be a psychiatrist. The only exception is for an emergency seventy-two-hour admission, when the written recommendation of one doctor is sufficient.

Crises

Mental health crises can happen at any time of the day or night. If you are very worried about the behaviour of some-one close to you, or perhaps afraid that they may do harm to themselves or others, your first step is to contact their GP. If you are unable to do this, or if the GP refuses to come out, then you can telephone your local social services depart-ment. Many have an out-of-hours emergency service; if so, and it is out of office hours ring the general emergency number for your local authority (which you will find in the telephone directory), and they will put you through. Alter-natively, the local police station will get in touch for you.

An Approved Social Worker is bound to visit if requested by a nearest relative. In most instances they will also visit or advise over the phone even if you are not the nearest relative although there is no obligation on them to do so.

If you are unable to get in touch either with the GP or social services you can take the person to the nearest hospital casualty department and ask to see the duty psychi-atrist; otherwise you could simply ring the hospital and ask for advice. As a last resort, in very serious circumstances, you could call in the police for assistance but you should be aware that this may result in the person being charged with an offence, if one has been committed.

If the Approved Social Worker is making the application for admission then he or she must interview the person concerned to find out about means of support both within the family and the community and how they feel about going into hospital on a voluntary basis, if appropriate. The aim is to see if there might be any possible alternatives to compulsory admission. If, however, it does seem the best means of providing the attention and care that is needed the person will then be examined by the doctors who will give their medical opinion.

The main grounds for compulsorily admission – which is always seen as a last resort – are that the individual is suffering from a mental disorder to a degree that warrants detention for either assessment or treatment and that he or she also needs to be detained in the interests of his or her own health or safety or for the protection of others.

There are various ways of compulsorily detaining a person depending on individual circumstances. Each is outlined under a different section of the Mental Health Act 1983. For convenience these methods are often simply referred to by their appropriate section numbers, which you may find a little confusing. You may also hear a compulsorily detained or formal patient referred to as a patient who has been sectioned or who is on a section. If you are not sure which section is being applied to you or your relative, always ask; it is your right to know. Incidentally, you may also be puzzled by references to the RMO, or Responsible Medical Officer; this is simply the term for the psychiatrist in charge of your case.

This chapter looks first at the situation for those patients detained and discharged under the civil sections in Part II of the Mental Health Act 1983.

Civil admission

Section 2 Patients can be detained for up to 28 days for assessment of their condition. Assessment is sometimes accompanied by treatment. An application for admission can be made by the Approved Social Worker without the nearest relative's consent.

Section 3 This section covers admission for treatment for up to six months. It can be renewed for a further six months, and then for periods of a year at a time by the psychiatrist in charge of the case after consultation with one or more people professionally concerned with the patient's medical treatment. Admission under this section needs the consent of the nearest relative. If the nearest relative refuses and the Approved Social Worker thinks this unreasonable, he or she can ask the County Court to decide whether the nearest relative should be displaced by someone who would agree to the application.

Section 4 Patients are admitted under Section 4 only in an emergency, for example if they are violent or suicidal. The admission, which is for a maximum of seventy-two hours, is to enable an assessment to be made and a decision taken on whether to admit for longer. An application for admission can be made by the Approved Social Worker without the nearest relative's consent. The person need only be examined by one doctor who must, however, confirm in writing that the admission is of urgent necessity, and that waiting for another doctor would cause undesirable delay.

Section 5 Voluntary patients are normally free to discharge themselves when they wish. However, sometimes this may appear inadvisable and certain staff then have holding powers under the Act. The doctor in charge of the patient or the deputy can sign a report detaining a voluntary in-patient for up to seventy-two hours to give time for decisions to be made. After that time has elapsed the patient becomes an informal patient again, unless detained under another section.

When it is not possible for the appropriate doctor to attend immediately a nurse with the requisite qualifications also has the power to prevent an informal patient from leaving hospital for up to six hours, or until the appropriate doctor can attend, if it appears necessary for the health or safety of the patient or for the protection of others.

Role of the police

Many people are uncertain about the role of the police in compulsory detention. This is outlined in Sections 135 and 136 of the Mental Health Act 1983. In certain circumstances the police have the power to take someone suspected of mental disorder to a place of safety for a maximum of seventy-two hours. This can be any suitable place where the occupier is willing to receive that person temporarily. In practice it is usually a hospital or, less ideally, a police station.

During this time the person should be examined by a doctor and interviewed by an Approved Social Worker and any appropriate arrangements for care or treatment should be made. However, once the examination and interview have taken place the person must be released unless another section is enforced.

Section 135 This section might be used when an Approved Social Worker is unable to gain access to someone thought to be suffering from a mental disorder if it was suspected that that person might be being neglected, ill-treated, inadequately supervised or living alone and unable to care for themselves. The Approved Social Worker would apply to a magistrate for a warrant which would authorize a police officer, accompanied by an Approved Social Worker and a doctor, to enter the person's home and remove him or her to a place of safety.

Section 136 This section applies to someone who appears to a police officer to be suffering from a mental disorder in a public place, and to be in immediate need of care and control. The police officer may take that person to a place of safety.

Civil discharge

When patients have completed the amount of time stipulated by the sections they are under they automatically become informal patients and are free to discharge themselves unless further measures are taken to continue their detention.

Patients, however, may be discharged before their section has ended by the psychiatrist in charge of their case, or the hospital managers, if it is agreed that the patient no longer needs to remain in hospital. Patients may be allowed home for trial periods by their psychiatrist while still on a section, but will, of course, be subject to recall.

In some circumstances the nearest relative can discharge a detained patient. If you have a relative detained under Section 2 or 3 and you are unhappy about this, first ask to speak to the psychiatrist in charge of the case. You can, as the nearest relative, apply to have the patient discharged by giving seventy-two hours notice in writing to the hospital managers if you are convinced this is the right thing to do. However, the psychiatrist in charge of the case can prevent the discharge through a report to the hospital managers giving reasons why the patient should be detained. As this procedure is so complex it would be sensible to take advice first from a Citizens Advice Bureau or from MIND's Legal and Welfare Rights Department (see Chapter 18).

Mental Health Review Tribunal

Another means' of discharge is through a Mental Health Review Tribunal. Patients under Section 2 and Section 3 can apply. So can the nearest relative of a patient under Section 3. Forms are available from the hospital administrative office or from the nearest Mental Health Review Tribunal Office (see addresses on pp. 205–6).

A Mental Health Review Tribunal is an independent body consisting of a lawyer, a psychiatrist – always from a hospital other than where the patient is detained – and a lay person with experience in the mental health field. The tribunal's task is to consider all the evidence and decide whether a patient should be discharged now or at some specified future date, or whether the decision should be left to the psychiatrist in charge of the case. Although this is an informal proceeding and not a court of law it does help to be represented. In most cases it is preferable that this should be by a solicitor, although in some cases it might be by someone such as an advice worker or friend you have confidence in.

You can obtain legal aid to pay for advice and representation by a solicitor if your income is below a certain level; the solicitor you select will deal with this for you. Legal aid will also pay for the cost of independent reports that may be needed. A list of lawyers trained in this type of work has been produced by the Law Society. You should be able to obtain it from the hospital administration office, from your local social services department or by writing to the Law Society direct (address on p. 208).

You cannot apply to a tribunal if you are only detained for seventy-two hours. However, if you are admitted under Section 2 for up to twenty-eight days you can apply during the first fourteen days, and your case must be heard within seven days. If you are admitted under Section 3 for up to six months you may apply at any time during your detention but unfortunately your case may not be heard as promptly as under Section 2. If your detention is renewed under Section 3 you may apply once more during the second six months and once during any subsequent year. If a patient does not apply under Section 3 in the first six months the case will automatically be referred to the tribunal if detention is renewed. Long-stay patients are automatically referred when three years have elapsed since their last hearing.

Criminal proceedings

Sections in Part III of the Mental Health Act 1983 may sometimes be used when people with mental illness are involved in criminal proceedings.

If you or a relative are suspected of committing a criminal offence and are or have been suffering from mental illness, then it is very important that you seek good legal advice and fully understand all the implications. Remember, your solicitor is working for you and should explain all the advantages and disadvantages of the various options open to you. Legal aid should be available, so check with your solicitor.

Evidence from doctors will be required if mental illness is to be taken into account by the court.

If it is apparent that you were suffering from mental illness at the time you were arrested, the Crown Prosecution Service may simply decide not to prosecute.

If you are judged to be suffering from mental illness at the time of the trial, you might be found unfit to plead and sent to hospital as if you were being detained under the Mental Health Act 1983.

You might also be remanded to hospital under Section 35 for up to twelve weeks to enable a report to be made on your condition to assist the court in reaching a decision about sentencing. This would be done only if there was thought to be no other practical way of obtaining the report on a voluntary out-patient or in-patient basis.

You could also be remanded to hospital for treatment under Section 36 for up to twelve weeks if it was considered appropriate.

If the court decides you were suffering from a mental disorder at the time of the offence, that may in certain circumstances amount to a defence. This is a very complicated area of law but your lawyer will advise you if you are in this situation.

If you are judged to be suffering from mental illness at the time of sentencing there are various possible outcomes. For example, you might be put on probation with a condition of psychiatric treatment, which means that you can receive treatment as an out-patient or voluntary in-patient. Alternatively, you might be compulsorily admitted to hospital under a hospital order (Section 37) for up to six months if the court thinks you will benefit from hospital admission and that this is the most suitable way to deal with your case. The order can be renewed for a further six months and then for a year at a time.

In certain circumstances a restriction order (Section 41) can accompany the hospital order. A restriction order is made if the court believes that this is necessary to protect the public 'from serious harm'. A patient on a restriction order can be discharged only by a Mental Health Review Tribunal or the Home Secretary. You may need legal advice on your rights.

Sometimes, when there is doubt as to whether a hospital order is appropriate, a patient may be detained under an interim hospital order (Section 38) for up to six months to enable a decision to be made.

Finally, if you are suffering from mental illness while awaiting trial in prison or serving a prison sentence, you can be transferred to hospital by the Home Secretary under the Mental Health Act, if this seems advisable.

Of course, you should also be prepared for the fact that for certain offences you might simply receive a prison sentence.

Guardianship

Under Section 7 of the Mental Health Act 1983, local social services departments can impose a guardianship order for up to six months, renewable for a further six months and then for periods of a year at a time. This means that some patients who require formal care can remain in the community and avoid compulsory admission to hospital.

An application for guardianship must be made by an Approved Social Worker or the nearest relative and supported by recommendations in writing from two doctors, one of whom must be a psychiatrist. The consent of the nearest relative should be obtained but if he or she objects the Approved Social Worker can apply to the County Court to see whether the nearest relative can be displaced.

The guardian appointed will either be the local social services department or someone appointed by them. The guardian has powers to insist that the patient should live in a specified place and attend specified places for occupation, training or medical treatment, though patients do have the right to refuse treatment. Patients are also required to ensure that the doctor, social worker or anyone else named by the guardian can visit them at home.

Under Section 37 the courts can impose a guardianship order with the same requirements as an alternative to prison or hospital where someone is found guilty of an offence, although this is rarely done.

You may be discharged from a guardianship order by the psychiatrist in charge of your case, the social services department, your nearest relative or a Mental Health Review Tribunal.

Mental Health Commissions

England and Wales

The Mental Health Act Commission is a special body set up in 1983 to protect the rights and interests of detained patients in England and Wales. If you are a detained patient or a relative of one and have a complaint, first follow the normal procedures (see Chapter 11). If you have done so and are still not satisfied, you can get in touch with the Commission (addresses on p. 206–7).

The Commission has a number of other functions and members of the Commission may visit you while you are detained. If so, you should be given the opportunity to air any grievances.

Scotland

The Mental Welfare Commission for Scotland (address on p. 207) performs a much wider function than the Mental Health Act Commission. It deals with complaints from all patients, whether detained or voluntary, as well as general inquiries on mental health problems and appeals for discharge from detained patients.

Northern Ireland

The Mental Health Commission in Northern Ireland (address on p. 207) also has a wider role than the Mental Health Act Commission. It can deal with the complaints of detained patients and it also has a duty to review the care and treatment of all mentally ill people, whether they are detained or voluntary patients in hospital, or living in the community.

CHAPTER 17

Commonly Confused Terms

Mental health problems are distressing enough without having to struggle with the meaning of words. Unfortunately, the mental health field abounds with names and terms that tend to confuse and mystify the lay person and thus cause additional anxiety.

Apart from difficulties in understanding the jargon, we may feel even more bewildered when we discover that in some instances the same word is used in a different sense by different professionals or that words we are accustomed to use in everyday speech have a rather different meaning in a mental health context. And, finally, the fact that so many words in the mental health field begin with the prefix 'psych', which comes from the Greek word 'psyche' meaning mind or soul, adds to the confusion.

Specialists in all fields are lazy about using terms and expecting others to understand them, and those in mental health are no exception. But there is no reason why you should be expected to comprehend their language. Always ask for explanations of any names or terms you do not understand and if the explanation is still unclear, ask for a concrete example. You will often find that words sound much less threatening once their meaning is apparent.

Professions starting with 'psych'

Psychiatrists, psychologists, psychotherapists and psychoanalysts are all involved in trying to help people sort out their mental health problems in their own particular way but most people are confused by the similarities in their names and are unclear about the differences in their roles.

Psychiatrist

The important thing to remember about a psychiatrist is that he or she is a qualified medical doctor with further training in diagnosing and treating mental health problems (see Chapter 7). Because they are doctors, psychiatrists can prescribe drugs or recommend other types of physical treatment, and they will usually give physical forms of treatment careful consideration when looking at the whole range of support and therapy available.

Psychologist

A psychologist is someone who has a degree in psychology, the study of human and animal behaviour. A clinical psychologist (see Chapter 7) has completed further training in the health field and has skills in assessing and treating certain mental health problems. He or she is not medically qualified, apart from in certain rare cases, and does not prescribe drugs. Treatments are usually drawn from a range of talking and behaviour-based therapies (see Chapters 9 and 10) and are usually fairly short term.

An educational psychologist (see Chapter 5) has an additional post-graduate qualification in educational psychology as well as a teaching qualification and a minimum of two years teaching experience. Most educational psychologists are employed by local education authorities and work in a number of schools, offering help where children have problems that seem to be related to school. They will work with the parents and teachers, as well as the child concerned, to try to sort out what the problem is and find an acceptable means of dealing with it.

Psychotherapist

Unfortunately, the term psychotherapist is a vague one. It may refer to someone who has completed a lengthy and highly regarded training or to a person who has had little training at all.

Psychotherapy is a talking treatment and the role of the psychotherapist is to help you explore your inner world and your early childhood experiences so that you can better understand your present feelings and reactions and feel more confident to deal with them (see Chapter 9).

Your psychotherapist will not prescribe drugs even if he or she happens to be a doctor. You may see a psychotherapist once or several times a week over a period of months or years. Even weekly visits over a short period may give you valuable insights about yourself and the impetus to change. With more frequent visits over longer periods, however, you will have both the time and support to look more deeply at yourself.

Psychoanalyst

A qualified psychoanalyst will have undergone a recognized, thorough and lengthy training, including a training analysis, in order to carry out the most intensive form of talking therapy. If you decide to have psychoanalysis, you would expect to see your analyst daily, or three times a week if he or she practises a form of analysis known as analytic psychotherapy, over a number of years.

At present analysis is available only in London and a few large cities and you are most unlikely to be offered it on the

NHS. It is a very expensive form of treatment, but there are occasionally places available with supervised trainee analysts at reduced rates. Ask your GP or psychiatrist.

Psychoanalysis, like psychotherapy, aims to help you understand the influences that your early childhood experiences and your inner, unconscious world exert on your present life. The unconscious is that part of your mind containing feelings, impulses, memories and images that you are not directly aware of, but which you may be able to tap through dreams or creative work, for example, or by letting your thoughts flow freely, a process known to analysts as free association.

Analysts believe it is particularly important to uncover those parts of your experience that you have shut off or repressed because they were too painful to cope with. Once you can face them and come to terms with them, you will have a greater sense of completeness and freedom. Seeing an analyst so frequently means that you will feel supported while you deal with these painful areas.

Transference, an important aspect of analysis, occurs when you transfer to your therapist many of your early emotions, such as anger, which you felt for your father or mother, for example, but did not express. You are then able to re-experience these feelings, which you were unaware of but which have continued to bubble beneath the surface, and work through them in a positive way so that they no longer sap your energy or impede your life.

Most people associate psychoanalysis with a couch. However, most analysts would offer you the option of sitting in a chair and would certainly not expect you to use a couch unless you felt happy to do so. However, many people do find that lying on a couch, with the analyst sitting behind them, cuts down on external distraction and helps them concentrate more fully on their inner world.

Psychosomatic

The word psychosomatic – derived from psyche, meaning mind, and soma, meaning body – is used to describe physical disorders that are thought to be largely caused or aggravated by emotional upset or psychological stress. A skin rash you have acquired in response to anxiety or a back pain that is a symptom of your depression, for example, may therefore be termed psychosomatic. It is well recognized that our minds and bodies interact extremely closely and that emotional and psychological factors play a part in many physical illnesses, just as physical illnesses in turn may affect our emotional and psychological well-being.

Unfortunately, the word psychosomatic has gained a rather dismissive meaning in everyday speech, as though people with psychosomatic complaints are being self-indulgent or as if their conditions are in some way less real. This, of course, is not the case. If your doctor tells you your symptoms are psychosomatic, it simply means that your body has responded in a physical way, which is outside your control, to feelings of stress, depression or anxiety, for example. You may therefore sometimes need help in dealing with your emotional or psychological difficulties before your physical symptoms can improve.

Psychoses and neuroses

There are some pairs of words in the mental health field that give the erroneous impression that people with mental health problems can be neatly categorized. One such pair you may come across is psychoses and neuroses, though these terms tend to be less widely used than formerly.

The psychoses, or psychotic disorders, refer to what are generally thought of as the more severe forms of mental disorder, such as manic-depression and schizophrenia (see

Chapters 3 and 4). People suffering from these so-called psychoses are considered to be unable to cope with the demands of ordinary life and are thought not to have insight into their own condition or to be aware that they need help. Their perceptions are distorted and they seem to lose contact with reality, so that they are unable to distinguish between what is actually happening in the outside world and what is going on in their own internal world of confused thoughts and feelings.

The term neuroses, or neurotic disorders, on the other hand, is generally applied to the less severe, although still distressing, disorders such as anxiety states, phobias, obsessions and some forms of depression where the person concerned generally has insight into the fact that something is wrong as well as a fairly rational view of the world.

The way 'neurotic' is used in a mental health context should not be confused with the way the word is used in ordinary language, when it is often a term of criticism for someone who is simply rather a worrier, or perhaps just a little tidier or more punctual than oneself.

Endogenous and reactive depression

There have been many attempts to classify depression into various types, or a number of different disorders, in the hope of understanding it better and making it easier to deal with. However, so far no classification has proved completely satisfactory, probably because so much still remains to be understood (see Chapter 2).

One classification you may hear referred to, for example, is the division into endogenous and reactive. Endogenous, which means coming from within, was originally used to refer to a depression that seemed to come out of the blue; it was attributed to changes occurring within the person rather than to any external cause. This type of depression has also been associated with a particular group of symptoms – including early morning waking, weight loss, slowing down in mind and body, and excessive guilt and self-reproach – which usually respond well to treatment with antidepressant drugs. Endogenous depression was sometimes also referred to as psychotic depression, though this did not necessarily mean that the person was out of touch with reality.

Reactive depression, sometimes also called neurotic depression, refers to a depression thought to result from an upsetting life event or personal difficulty and characterized by symptoms such as anxiety and tension.

However, it has become apparent that depression is more complex and the differences between types less clear-cut than previously supposed, and so the terms endogenous and reactive are now less widely used.

Mental handicap and mental illness

Although mental illness and mental handicap are quite different conditions, many people are unclear about the distinction between them.

Mental handicap is the term for a number of different disorders in which the function of the brain is impaired so that it does not develop normally. This may occur before birth, during birth or sometimes after birth, through accident, illness or injury. Mental handicap is a permanent disability for which there is no treatment or cure, though a great deal can usually be achieved through education, training and support to enable people with mental handicap to make the most of their abilities and lead successful lives within the community. Obviously the more severe the handicap, the more support people will need. Of course, people with mental handicap are just as likely as anyone else to suffer from mental health problems.

Mental illness is the general term for a range of different disorders that affect the mind so that people previously able to cope with life are no longer able to do so. Mental illnesses can often be treated or alleviated, and they may sometimes improve of their own accord. In many cases such illnesses are only brief episodes; in others the effects are longer term.

Schizophrenia

One of the most widely misunderstood words in mental health is schizophrenia. It is quite frequently and wrongly used to refer to a split or multiple personality of the Jekyll and Hyde variety. Such a rapid switch from one complete personality type to a totally different one is rare and has nothing to do with schizophrenia. When it does occur, it is known as 'hysteric split personality' by those in the mental health professions. To confuse the issue further the word schizophrenic is now often used very loosely, and even flippantly, in everyday language to describe people who hold two different views at once, a far more common occurrence.

The word schizophrenia is derived from Greek words meaning split mind, though split in this sense refers to disintegration rather than a division into two parts. Schizophrenia is the name for a distressing mental illness or group of illnesses where the mind has difficulty in functioning as a whole and retaining its grasp on reality (see Chapter 4).

Nervous breakdown

'Nervous breakdown' is not a term that is often used by professionals in the mental health field since it has no exact meaning. However, it is often used by non-professionals to describe an episode of mental distress in which a person is no longer able to cope and needs a complete rest or change of scene. To the casual observer, the onset of this state may appear as quite sudden, triggered off by a comparatively minor incident, but in fact the stresses may have been building up for a considerable time.

There are many different causes of so-called breakdowns, from overwork to the onset of a more serious psychiatric illness, and symptoms may range from shaking and tearfulness, for example, to delusions and hallucinations. Some breakdowns are relatively mild and recovery takes place after a few weeks' holiday; others are more serious and may even necessitate a stay in hospital. It is, therefore, clear that the term 'nervous breakdown' tells us very little, in fact, about a person's state.

CHAPTER 18

Resources

Although health and local authorities should aim to provide appropriate care and support for people with mental health problems, provision throughout the country is very uneven and there are many gaps. A well-developed scheme in one area may be unheard of in another and many services, when they do exist, are overstretched. Support for relatives is similarly patchy.

If you or a relative are struggling to cope with a mental health problem you may have to be quite persistent to get the help you want. Quite often voluntary organizations can offer advice or assistance, while a telephone help-line or self-help group can provide essential support. However, you do need information on what exists so that you can make the best use of what is available.

This chapter describes some organizations that can either offer help themselves or refer you to other sources of help. It is by no means a comprehensive list but it should give you a good start. Addresses of useful law organizations are also listed.

One advantage of looking for help yourself in this way is that it enables you to feel that you are doing something constructive at a time when your confidence may be rather low. Another is that you may find there is more choice in the type of support available than you had originally thought.

General sources of help

Citizens Advice Bureaux (CAB)

Anyone can use a CAB. The service is free and confidential. Trained CAB workers offer information and advice on a wide range of subjects, including benefits, debts, housing, consumer, employment and legal problems, and family and personal difficulties. Your CAB should have details of useful local services and organizations, including self-help groups and counselling agencies, as well as national organizations. Ask for the address of your nearest CAB at the library or look in the telephone book. Check on opening times, as these vary.

Community Health Councils (CHC)

CHCs represent the interests of the consumer in the health service. There is at least one to each health district. Contact your local CHC for information on local NHS services and your entitlements, and for assistance if you wish to make a complaint. CHCs should be able to advise you if you are experiencing difficulties with some aspect of the NHS. They should also be able to tell you about other helpful organizations and groups, and may assist in setting up self-help groups. CHCs are listed in the telephone book under 'Community', or under the name of your district health authority. In Scotland they are known as Local Health Councils, and in Northern Ireland as District Committees. Opening times vary.

Councils for Voluntary Service

These councils, or their equivalent, can give information about voluntary organizations in your area. They can also assist in setting up self-help and support groups. They are usually listed in the telephone book under Council for

Voluntary Service, or a similar title, or under the name of the area. You can telephone or write to them for information.

Family Practitioner Committee (FPC)

Everyone is entitled to be registered with a doctor. If you are new to an area, you will find lists of local doctors at the local FPC, Community Health Council or Citizens Advice Bureau (the addresses are in the telephone book), but probably the best way is to ask friends and neighbours. If you have difficulty in finding a doctor to take you, inform the FPC. They will ensure that you get one.

If you wish to change your doctor, first find another GP who is willing to take you on. Then either inform your own doctor, who should sign your medical card, or send your card to the FPC telling them of your wish to change. You do not have to give a reason. This procedure takes about fourteen days.

For advice on getting or changing a doctor in Scotland, contact your local Health Board; the address is in the telephone book. In Northern Ireland, write to:
Central Services Agency
25–27 Adelaide Street
Belfast
BT2 8FH

Local advice agencies

There may be a number of useful agencies in your area offering advice on a number of topics, or specializing, for example, in law or housing. To find out what exists, ask at your library or the town hall.

Places of religious worship

If you attend a place of worship, apart from the strength that you may gain from your faith, various forms of support may be available. You should not be embarrassed to ask. Many religious organizations offer counselling, support groups and practical assistance. There may also be specific charities connected with your religion that can offer help.

Private health care

If your GP suggests you see a psychiatrist and you have private medical insurance, you may wish to check whether you are covered for private psychiatric consultation and treatment as an in- or out-patient, and if so, to what extent. If you are claiming on insurance, then you must be referred by your GP to a consultant psychiatrist. (Private medical insurance offers only very limited cover, if any, for psychotherapy.) If you are paying out of your own pocket, you can refer yourself, though it is always sensible to discuss this with your GP, if possible.

You are not likely to be offered different or better treatment privately, but you are likely to be seen more quickly and in more comfortable surroundings. You will also be seen by the consultant psychiatrist on each occasion and not by a junior doctor.

Public libraries

Your local library is often a starting point for finding out addresses of local and national organizations. It may also have information about informal local clubs and societies, sports and recreational activities, day and evening classes and holiday schemes, which can help you make the best use of what is available in your area. Librarians are usually helpful in feretting out information or pointing you in the right direction.

Social Security Freeline

Trained staff from the Department of Social Security offer advice and information on benefits over the telephone, free of charge to callers; this is a particularly useful service for busy or housebound people. Telephone 0800–666555 between 8 a.m. and 6 p.m. weekdays if you live in England, Scotland or Wales. Northern Ireland has an equivalent service; telephone 0800–616757 between 9 a.m. and 4.30 p.m. weekdays.

Social services

Many people do not realize that they can ring the social services department direct for information and advice, or for support or practical help. All social services departments have social workers who are particularly experienced in mental health. They can tell you what social services can offer, and what else is available in the area. Contact them to find out about facilities such as day centres and other daytime activities, residential accommodation, home helps, meals on wheels, aids and adaptations.

If you are particularly worried about your own situation or that of someone in your family, you can ask to see a social worker to talk things through. You can telephone or call in. You can contact an Approved Social Worker for help in a crisis (see Chapter 16). Social services are listed in the phone book under the name of your local authority.

Volunteer Bureaux

Volunteer Bureaux throughout the UK train and support volunteers to work in the community with organizations or individuals. If you as a carer would like a volunteer to help you perhaps once or twice a week – so that you can do your shopping or have some time to yourself, for example – contact your local bureau. You will have the opportunity to interview a volunteer and see whether he or she would be appropriate. If no one suitable is available, your name will go on a waiting list.

If on the other hand you are recovering from mental health problems but are not yet ready to return to paid employment, you may wish to contribute to the community through voluntary work. Contact your local bureau to see if there is a suitable project you could take part in. Some bureaux run specific projects for volunteers who need extra support. Volunteer Bureaux can also put you in touch with other local voluntary organizations and self-help groups. Look under Volunteer Bureau in your local telephone directory, or telephone or write to:

National Association of Volunteer Bureaux
St Peter's College
College Road
Saltley, Birmingham B8 37E
Tel: 021–327–02650

Specialized Sources of Help

Age Concern

Local Age Concern groups throughout the UK provide services for elderly people and their carers with the help of volunteers. Each group is independent and activities vary, often depending on what other services are available locally. Age Concern groups may organize day-care centres, lunch clubs, over-60s clubs, visits to the housebound, sitting-in services and relative support groups, as well as offering advice and information on rights, benefits and other local organizations and services. To find your nearest group look in the telephone book under Age Concern or ask at the library.

Alcohol problems

Alcoholics Anonymous (AA) AA is a network of independent self-help groups. Members encourage each other to stop drinking and to stay off drink through mutual support at meetings and at other times. Anonymity is preserved by the use of first names. To contact your nearest group, look in the telephone book or write or telephone:

AA General Service Office
  PO Box 1
  Stonebow House
  Stonebow, York YO1 2NJ
  Tel: 0904–644026

Al-Anon and Alateen Al-Anon Family Groups provide support and information for relatives and close friends of problem drinkers, whether or not the drinker is also seeking help. Alateen, which is part of Al-Anon, offers support to teenagers whose lives have been affected by an alcoholic friend or relative. For information on your nearest local group, write or telephone the central office, which also provides a 24-hour confidential helpline service manned by members.

Al-Anon Family Groups
  61 Great Dover Street
  London SE1 4YF
  Tel: 01–403–0888

Alcohol Concern For information on alcohol problems, what type of services exist and where you can get help, in England and Wales, write to or telephone:

Alcohol Concern
  305 Gray's Inn Road
  London WC1X 8QF
  Tel: 01–833–3471

In Scotland contact:
    Scottish Council on Alcohol
    137–145 Sauchiehall Street
    Glasgow GT 3EN
    Tel: 041–333–9677
In Northern Ireland contact:
    Council on Alcohol
    40 Elmwood Avenue
    Belfast BT9 6AZ
    Tel: 0232–664434

Alzheimer's Disease Society

This organization supports carers of those suffering from Alzheimer's and other forms of dementia. Contact the society for information on Alzheimer's and related illnesses, advice on services available and details of your nearest local support group.

If you live in England, Wales or Northern Ireland, write or telephone:
Alzheimer's Disease Society
    158/160 Balham High Road
    London SW12 9BN
    Tel: 01–675–6557/8/9/0
If you live in Scotland, contact:
Alzheimer's Scotland
    1st Floor
    40 Shandwick Place
    Edinburgh EH2 4RT
    Tel: 031–225–1453/6367

Anorexic Family Aid

This national information centre on anorexia and bulimia provides information on treatment available in the UK, helpful guidelines and a telephone helpline for sufferers, friends and relatives during office hours. It can also put you in touch with local self-help groups. It has now merged with Anorexic Aid and will in future be known as Eating Disorders Association. Write or telephone:

Anorexic Family Aid Information Centre
   Sackville Place
   44–48 Magdalen Street
   Norwich, Norfolk NR3 1JE
   Tel: 0603–621414

British Association for Counselling (BAC)

The BAC has a list of counsellors, some of whom are accredited by the BAC, as well as of counselling and psychotherapy organizations throughout the UK. Write, enclosing a stamped, addressed envelope, to:

British Association for Counselling
   37a Ship Street
   Rugby, Warwickshire CU21 3BX

Carers National Association

Carers exists to support people whose lives may be restricted by caring for someone who has mental health problems, a mental or physical handicap or who is elderly or infirm. It encourages carers to recognize that their needs are as important as those of the people they are caring for, and campaigns for greater resources for carers and greater understanding of their role. It answers queries from carers in the UK by letter or phone and acts as an initial counselling service for those who are desperate. It offers information on services and benefits and can put people in touch with local sources of help and with local carers' support groups or assist in the setting up of such a group. Write or telephone:

Carers National Association
  29 Chilworth Mews
  London W2 3RG
  Tel: 01–724–7776

Children

Association for Post-Natal Illness The association provides leaflets and a network of telephone and postal volunteers in the UK who have themselves experienced post-natal illness and who can offer support and encouragement on a one-to-one basis. Write, enclosing a stamped, addressed envelope, to:
Association for Post-Natal Illness
  7 Gowan Avenue
  Fulham
  London SW6 6RH

Gingerbread Bringing up children on your own can be rewarding, but it can also be lonely and stressful. Gingerbread is an association for one-parent families. It has a large network of self-help groups, which offer information, support and an opportunity to enjoy family activities with others. For information, literature or the address of your nearest group, write or telephone:
Gingerbread
  35 Wellington Street
  London WC2E 7BN
  Tel: 01–240–0953

MAMA If you feel lonely at home looking after children, Meet a Mum Association will try to put you in touch with another mother nearby or a group of mothers, if one exists

locally, or help you find ways of meeting people. Write or telephone:
MAMA,
  5 Westbury Gardens
  Luton
  Beds LU2 7DW
  Tel: 0582-422253

National Council for One-Parent Families The council has an advice department that can help you deal with practical matters ranging from financial and legal problems to child care and housing or refer you to appropriate organizations.

In England, Wales or Northern Ireland write or telephone on any weekday except Wednesday:
National Council for One-Parent Families
  255 Kentish Town Road
  London NW5 2LX
  Tel: 01–267–1361
In Scotland, contact:
The Scottish Council for Single Parents
  13 Gayfield Square
  Edinburgh EH1 3NX
  Tel: 031–556–3899

Cruse-Bereavement Care

This national organization offers advice and counselling to bereaved people. They can put you in touch with a local branch, if one exists in your area, or help you directly. Local branches may run groups, which can be a first step to overcoming loneliness. Cruse also works closely with other organizations helping bereaved people. Write or telephone:
Cruse-Bereavement Care
  126 Sheen Road
  Richmond, Surrey TW9 1UR
  Tel: 01–940–4818

Depressives Anonymous

This is a self-help organization for past and present sufferers from depression. It publishes a quarterly newsletter, organizes open meetings and a pen-friend scheme and can put you in touch with a local self-help group, if one exists in your area, or advise on starting one. Write, enclosing a stamped, addressed envelope, or telephone:

The Fellowship of Depressives Anonymous
36 Chestnut Avenue
Beverley, North Humberside HU17 9QU
Tel: 0482–860619

Depressives Associated

This organization provides information on depression and suggestions for coping for sufferers and relatives. It will try to put sufferers in touch with a local self-help group, if one exists, or with other individuals in the area, and it operates a pen-friend scheme. Write to:

Depressives Associated
PO Box 5
Castletown
Portland, Dorset DT5 1BQ

Drug problems

Narcotics Anonymous Members of this self-help organization for addicts help each other stay clear of drugs through a helpline and local support groups. Write or telephone between 12 p.m. and 8 p.m. for information on your nearest local group or counselling. All calls are answered by drug-free recovering addicts, who will understand your worries.

Narcotics Anonymous
PO Box 417
London SW10 0DP
Tel: 01–351–6794/6066

Families Anonymous This organization offers support through a helpline and self-help groups to the families and friends of those with a drug or drug-related behaviour problem to help them find ways of better coping with this difficult situation. The telephone is manned by members who have been through similar situations and will understand your anxiety. Write or telephone:

Families Anonymous
310 Finchley Road
London NW3 7AG
Tel: 01–731–8060

SCODA These are the initials of the Standing Conference on Drug Abuse, which provides information on local treatment and services to help drug users, family and friends throughout the UK. Write to:

SCODA
1–4 Hatton Place
London EC1 8ND

For information on services in England and Wales, you can also ask the operator for Freefone Drug Problems. This will give you a contact number for your area.

For information on services in Scotland, you can also write or telephone:

Scottish Drugs Forum
266 Clyde Street
Glasgow G1 4JH
Tel: 041–221–1175

Tranx This organization offers advice and support by letter, telephone or a walk-in service during office hours to people attempting to come off minor tranquillizers. Tranx will also put you in touch with a local self-help group, if one exists in your area. Contact:

Tranx
　25a Masons Avenue
　Wealdstone
　Harrow, Middlesex HA3 5AH
　Tel: 01–427–2065

Family Planning Information Service (FPIS)

Worries over any aspect of sex, including performance, sexual orientation, sexually transmitted diseases, fertility and contraception, can lead to anxiety, depression or relationship difficulties, which can, in turn, affect confidence. If you are unable to discuss such a worry openly with your GP, you can contact the FPIS. It provides information on a range of sexual problems, which in itself may prove reassuring, and can suggest whom you should contact for further help and advice. Write, enclosing a stamped, addressed envelope, or telephone:
Family Planning Information Service
　27 Mortimer Street
　London W1N 7RJ
　Tel: 01–636–7866

Manic-Depression Fellowship

This is a self-help organization for sufferers and relatives. It organizes open meetings, produces a newsletter and puts people in touch with local groups, where they exist, or advises on setting them up. Write to:
Manic-Depression Fellowship
　51 Sheen Road
　Richmond, Surrey TW9 1YQ
　Tel: 01–332–1078 (messages only)

Mental Health Associations

MIND, National Association for Mental Health MIND campaigns for better mental health services throughout England

and Wales. Through its national headquarters, its regional offices and its network of around 200 local groups, MIND works to combat the stigma that still surrounds the term 'mental illness', as well as to uphold the rights and represent the views of people with mental health problems and increase the understanding of mental health throughout the community.

You can write or telephone National MIND for advice and information relating to mental health problems. If the problem relates specifically to legal or welfare rights, contact the Legal and Welfare Rights Department, preferably by letter. Contact the Advice Unit for advice about mental health problems, and the Information Unit for information on all aspects of mental health. MIND publishes a range of books and leaflets.

National MIND
    22 Harley Street
    London W1N 2ED
    Tel: 01–637–0741

Contact your Regional MIND office for information about its campaigning activities, services and helpful voluntary organizations in your area, and for the address of your local MIND group.

North-west MIND
    21 Ribblesdale Place
    Preston PR1 3NA
    Tel: 0772–21734

Northern MIND
    158 Durham Road
    Gateshead NE8 4EL
    Tel: 091–490–0109

Wales MIND
    23 St Mary Street
    Cardiff CF1 2AA
    Tel: 0222–395123

South-east MIND
  4th Floor
  24–32 Stephenson Way
  London NW1 2HD
  Tel: 01–380–1253
South-west MIND
  9th Floor, Tower House
  Fairfax Street
  Bristol BS1 3BN
  Tel: 0272–250960
West Midlands MIND
  20–21 Cleveland Street
  Wolverhampton WV1 3HT
  Tel: 0902–24404
Trent and Yorkshire MIND
  The White Building
  Fitzalan Square
  Sheffield S1 2AY
  Tel: 0742–21742

Contact your local MIND group to see what it can offer you, since activities vary considerably. You may wish to join. As well as campaigning locally for better services, it may offer support through information and advice services, befriending schemes, employment projects or self-help groups, for example. It may also provide services to complement those offered by local authorities, such as supported housing schemes, drop-in centres and social clubs. All local groups should be able to point you in the right direction for other services.

Scottish Association for Mental Health (SAMH) SAMH is the Scottish equivalent of MIND and campaigns for better mental health services and an increased understanding of mental health in Scotland. It provides information on mental health issues and can direct you to relevant services, organizations and self-help groups in your area, as well as to local associations for mental health. SAMH is also closely involved in projects to provide employment and accommodation. Ring, write or call in at:

Scottish Association for Mental Health
   Atlantic House
   38 Gardeners Crescent
   Edinburgh EH3 8DP
   Tel: 031–229–9687

Activities of local associations vary; they may include local support groups, counselling, social clubs, drop-in and day centres and accommodation projects.

Northern Ireland Association for Mental Health (NIAMH)

NIAMH is the Northern Ireland equivalent of MIND and has the same broad aims. It offers advice and information on mental health issues and can direct you to local services, organizations and self-help groups in your area as well as to local branches. It also runs a free drop-in service one evening a week where people can talk to professionals about any mental health problem. Ring, write or call in at:

Northern Ireland Association for Mental Health
   84 University Street
   Belfast BT7 1HE
   Tel: 0232–328474

Activities of local branches vary, but all include Beacon House social clubs. Some run self-help groups, day centres and acommodation projects.

National Schizophrenia Fellowship

This organization offers information, advice and support to friends and relatives of people with schizophrenia and related problems, and to the people themselves. It can also put relatives in touch with local self-help groups; these provide mutual support and are sometimes also actively involved in local projects. Telephone or write:

National Schizophrenia Fellowship
Head Office
  78 Victoria Road
  Surbiton, Surrey KT6 4NS
  Tel: 01–390–3651
National Schizophrenia Fellowship (Scotland)
  40 Shandwick Place
  Edinburgh EH2 4RT
  Tel: 031–226–2025
National Schizophrenia Fellowship (Northern Ireland)
  Regional Office
  47 Rosemary Street
  Belfast BT1 1QB
  Tel: 0232–248006

Phobics Society

This is the national society for sufferers from all types of phobia and obsessional neurosis. It offers help and information and provides a list of members willing to be contacted who can both listen and share their own experiences. Write, enclosing a stamped, addressed envelope, or telephone during office hours:

Phobics Society
  4 Cheltenham Road
  Chorlton-cum-Hardy
  Manchester M21 1QN
  Tel: 061–881–1937

Relate: Marriage Guidance (formerly Marriage Guidance)

If you and your partner are experiencing stresses that you are unable to sort out together, you may find it helpful to talk to a Relate counsellor with your partner or on your own. Relate counsellors are carefully trained volunteers who will listen to you without making judgements. Their aim will be to help you sort out what you really feel so that you can look more clearly at your situation and work out the best course of action for yourself.

The address of your nearest Relate: Marriage Guidance council is in the telephone book; look under both Relate and Marriage Guidance. You do not have to be married to contact them. Telephone or write for an appointment, preferably before crisis point, as there is usually a one- to two-month wait, or longer. Counselling sessions take an hour and are on a weekly basis, lasting on average from six to eight weeks. You will be asked for a donation if you can afford it.

Samaritans

Samaritans are there to listen to your pain and distress. They provide a totally confidential 24-hour telephone service, seven days a week and so are always available to offer emotional support to those for whom life may be getting too much to bear. You may find it a tremendous relief simply to talk to someone about your innermost feelings and difficulties, knowing that they will not make judgements or offer their own solutions. Anonymity can be preserved by using first names or no names, if you prefer. You can telephone the Samaritans at any time, or write or drop in at most centres during the day and evening. They are listed under Samaritans in the telephone book.

Self-help and support groups

These provide the opportunity for people who have undergone similar experiences to exchange ideas and information and offer each other mutual support. Some groups are organized for people with specific mental health problems, some for relatives or carers and some are mixed.

Self-help groups are run by the members to meet their own needs. Support groups, on the other hand, may be run by a professional in the mental health field for people who share the same type of problem. Some groups will be free; others may ask for a contribution, usually to cover expenses.

To find out if there is a suitable self-help or support group in your area, ask your local Council for Voluntary Service, Community Health Council, Citizens Advice Bureau, GP surgery or hospital. If a suitable group does not exist and you have the energy to start one yourself, your local Council for Voluntary Service, Volunteer Bureau or Community Health Council should be able to advise you on how to set one up.

Survivors Speak Out

This national organization exists to promote the voice of the consumer in mental health services and campaign for a greater choice in care. It tries to put people in touch with local groups, where these exist, so that they can use their experience of mental health problems to advantage in working for better services, while at the same time giving each other support. Write or telephone:
Secretary
Survivors Speak Out
  33 Lichfield Road
  London NW2 2RJ
  Tel: 01–450–4631

Therapeutic communities

When someone has a mental health problem, particularly a young person, it is sometimes helpful if he or she can move

away to a supported environment and gradually gain independence. Therapeutic communities, usually run by registered charities, can act as a useful half-way house. They
offer the opportunity for people with mental health problems to live together and support each other with the help
of trained staff, and gradually take on more responsibility
for their own lives.

Communities vary, but most have regular group meetings
to discuss daily activities as well as personal and emotional
problems. Most people will stay from six months to two
years. Communities work closely with health and social
services, and funding is available for most residents. To find
out about therapeutic communities in your area ask your
GP, psychiatrist or social services or contact your regional
MIND office (see pp. 199–200).

The Richmond Fellowship runs a network of therapeutic
communities. For information contact:

Richmond Fellowship
  8 Addison Road
  London W14 6DL
  Tel: 01–603–6373

Legal addresses

Mental Health Review Tribunals (MHRT)

You can contact the MHRT nearest to the hospital through
the hospital administrative staff, the social worker or direct.
The addresses are:

  15th Floor
  Euston Tower
  286 Euston Road
  London NW1 3DN
  Tel: 01–388–1188, extension 3785/6/7

3rd Floor
Cressington House
249 St Mary's Road
Garston, Liverpool L19 0NF
Tel: 051–494–0095

Spur A
Block 5
Government Buildings
Chalfont Drive
Western Boulevard
Nottingham NG8 3RZ
Tel: 0602–294222

2nd Floor
New Crown Buildings
Cathays Park
Cardiff CF1 3NQ
Tel: 0222–825328

Northern Ireland Mental Health Review Tribunal
Room 112B
Dundonald House
Upper Newtownards Road
Belfast BT4 3SF
Tel: 02318–5550

Mental Health Act Commission
Contact the address nearest the hospital.
Floors 1 and 2
Hepburn House
Marsham Street
London SW1P 4HW
Tel: 01–217–6012/3

Cressington House
249 St Mary's Road
Garston, Liverpool L19 0NF
Tel: 051–427–2061

3rd Floor
Maid Marian House
Houndsgate, Nottingham NG1 6BG
Tel: 0602–410304

Mental Health Commission for Northern Ireland
Elizabeth House
116–118 Holywood Road
Belfast BT4 1NY
Tel: 0232–651157

Mental Welfare Commission for Scotland
25 Drumsheugh Gardens
Edinburgh EH3 7RB
Tel: 031–225–7034

Court of Protection
Stewart House
24 Kingsway
London WC2B 6JX
Tel: 01–269–7000

Office of Care and Protection
Royal Courts of Justice
Belfast BT1 3JF
Tel: 0232–235111

Law Society
Legal Practice Directorate
113 Chancery Lane
London WC2A 1PL
Tel: 01–242–1222

Law Society (Northern Ireland)
98 Victoria Street
Belfast BT1 3JZ
Tel: 0232–231614

Children's Legal Centre
20 Compton Terrace
London N1 2UN
Tel: 01–359–6251

INDEX

Discover more about our forthcoming books through Penguin's FREE newspaper...

Penguin

Quarterly

It's packed with:

- exciting features
- author interviews
- previews & reviews
- books from your favourite films & TV series
- exclusive competitions & much, much more...

Write off for your free copy today to:
Dept JC
Penguin Books Ltd
FREEPOST
West Drayton
Middlesex
UB7 0BR
NO STAMP REQUIRED

READ MORE IN PENGUIN

In every corner of the world, on every subject under the sun, Penguin represents quality and variety – the very best in publishing today.

For complete information about books available from Penguin – including Puffins, Penguin Classics and Arkana – and how to order them, write to us at the appropriate address below. Please note that for copyright reasons the selection of books varies from country to country.

In the United Kingdom: Please write to *Dept. JC, Penguin Books Ltd, FREEPOST, West Drayton, Middlesex UB7 OBR*

If you have any difficulty in obtaining a title, please send your order with the correct money, plus ten per cent for postage and packaging, to *PO Box No. 11, West Drayton, Middlesex UB7 OBR*

In the United States: Please write to *Penguin USA Inc., 375 Hudson Street, New York, NY 10014*

In Canada: Please write to *Penguin Books Canada Ltd, 10 Alcorn Avenue, Suite 300, Toronto, Ontario M4V 3B2*

In Australia: Please write to *Penguin Books Australia Ltd, 487 Maroondah Highway, Ringwood, Victoria 3134*

In New Zealand: Please write to *Penguin Books (NZ) Ltd,182–190 Wairau Road, Private Bag, Takapuna, Auckland 9*

In India: Please write to *Penguin Books India Pvt Ltd, 706 Eros Apartments, 56 Nehru Place, New Delhi 110 019*

In the Netherlands: Please write to *Penguin Books Netherlands B.V., Keizersgracht 231 NL–1016 DV Amsterdam*

In Germany: Please write to *Penguin Books Deutschland GmbH, Friedrichstrasse 10–12, W–6000 Frankfurt/Main 1*

In Spain: Please write to *Penguin Books S. A., C. San Bernardo 117–6° E–28015 Madrid*

In Italy: Please write to *Penguin Italia s.r.l., Via Felice Casati 20, I–20124 Milano*

In France: Please write to *Penguin France S. A., 17 rue Lejeune, F–31000 Toulouse*

In Japan: Please write to *Penguin Books Japan, Ishikiribashi Building, 2–5–4, Suido, Tokyo 112*

In Greece: Please write to *Penguin Hellas Ltd, Dimocritou 3, GR–106 71 Athens*

In South Africa: Please write to *Longman Penguin Southern Africa (Pty) Ltd, Private Bag X08, Bertsham 2013*

READ MORE IN PENGUIN

A SELECTION OF HEALTH BOOKS

The Kind Food Guide   Audrey Eyton

Audrey Eyton's all-time bestselling *The F-Plan Diet* turned the nation on to fibre-rich food. Now, as the tide turns against factory farming, she provides the guide destined to bring in a new era of eating.

Baby and Child   Penelope Leach

A beautifully illustrated and comprehensive handbook on the first five years of life. 'It stands head and shoulders above anything else available at the moment' – Mary Kenny in the *Spectator*

Woman's Experience of Sex   Sheila Kitzinger

Fully illustrated with photographs and line drawings, this book explores the riches of women's sexuality at every stage of life. 'A book which any mother could confidently pass on to her daughter – and her partner too' – *Sunday Times*

A Guide to Common Illnesses   Dr Ruth Lever

The complete, up-to-date guide to common complaints and their treatment, from causes and symptoms to cures, explaining both orthodox and complementary approaches.

Living with Alzheimer's Disease and Similar Conditions
Dr Gordon Wilcock

This complete and compassionate self-help guide is designed for families and carers (professional or otherwise) faced with the 'living bereavement' of dementia.

Living with Stress
Cary L. Cooper, Rachel D. Cooper and Lynn H. Eaker

Stress leads to more stress, and the authors of this helpful book show why low levels of stress are desirable and how best we can achieve them in today's world. Looking at those most vulnerable, they demonstrate ways of breaking the vicious circle that can ruin lives. .

READ MORE IN PENGUIN

A SELECTION OF HEALTH BOOKS

Living with Asthma and Hay Fever   John Donaldson

For the first time, there are now medicines that can prevent asthma attacks from taking place. Based on up-to-date research, this book shows how the majority of sufferers can beat asthma and hay fever to lead full and active lives.

Anorexia Nervosa   R. L. Palmer

Lucid and sympathetic guidance for those who suffer from this disturbing illness and their families and professional helpers, given with a clarity and compassion that will make anorexia more understandable and consequently less frightening for everyone involved.

Medical Treatments: Benefits and Risks   Peter Parish

The ultimate reference guide to the drug treatments available today – from over-the-counter remedies to drugs given under close medical supervision – for every common disease or complaint from acne to worms.

Pregnancy and Childbirth   Sheila Kitzinger
Revised Edition

A complete and up-to-date guide to physical and emotional preparation for pregnancy – a must for all prospective parents.

Miscarriage   Ann Oakley, Ann McPherson and Helen Roberts

One million women worldwide become pregnant every day. At least half of these pregnancies end in miscarriage or stillbirth. But each miscarriage is the loss of a potential baby, and that loss can be painful to adjust to. Here is sympathetic support and up-to-date information on one of the commonest areas of women's reproductive experience.

The Parents' A-Z   Penelope Leach

For anyone with children of 6 months, 6 years or 16 years, this guide to all the little problems in their health, growth and happiness will prove reassuring and helpful.

READ MORE IN PENGUIN

A SELECTION OF HEALTH BOOKS

When a Woman's Body Says No to Sex   Linda Valins

Vaginismus – an involuntary spasm of the vaginal muscles that prevents penetration – has been discussed so little that many women who suffer from it don't recognize their condition by its name. Linda Valins's practical and compassionate guide will liberate these women from their fears and sense of isolation and help them find the right form of therapy.

Medicine   The Self-Help Guide
Professor Michael Orme and Dr Susanna Grahame-Jones

A new kind of home doctor – with an entirely new approach. With a unique emphasis on self-management, *Medicine* takes an active approach to drugs, showing how to maximize their benefits, speed up recovery and minimize dosages through self-help and non-drug alternatives.

Defeating Depression   Tony Lake

Counselling, medication, and the support of friends can all provide invaluable help in relieving depression. But if we are to combat it once and for all, we must face up to perhaps painful truths about our past and take the first steps forward that can eventually transform our lives. This lucid and sensitive book shows us how.

Freedom and Choice in Childbirth   Sheila Kitzinger

Undogmatic, honest and compassionate, Sheila Kitzinger's book raises searching questions about the kind of care offered to the pregnant woman – and will help her make decisions and communicate effectively about the kind of birth experience she desires.

Care of the Dying   Richard Lamerton

It is never true that 'nothing more can be done' for the dying. This book shows us how to face death without pain, with humanity, with dignity and in peace.

READ MORE IN PENGUIN

A SELECTION OF HEALTH BOOKS

Twins, Triplets and More Elizabeth Bryan

This enlightening study of the multiple birth phenomenon covers all aspects of the subject from conception and birth to old age and death. It also offers much comfort and support as well as carefully researched information gained from meeting several thousands of children and their families.

Meditation for Everybody Louis Proto

Meditation is liberation from stress, anxiety and depression. This lucid and readable book by the author of *Self-Healing* describes a variety of meditative practices. From simple breathing exercises to more advanced techniques, there is something here to suit everybody's needs.

Endometriosis Suzie Hayman

Endometriosis is currently surrounded by many damaging myths. Suzie Hayman's pioneering book will set the record straight and provide both sufferers and their doctors with the information necessary for an improved understanding of this frequently puzzling condition.

My Child Won't Eat Nick Yapp

Written by a qualified nutritionist, this reassuring guide will provide parents with the facts, help and comfort that will put their minds at rest and allow them to feed their children with confidence.

Not On Your Own Sally Burningham
The MIND Guide to Mental Health

Cutting through the jargon and confusion surrounding the subject of mental health to provide clear explanations and useful information, *Not On Your Own* will enable those with problems – as well as their friends and relatives – to make the best use of available help or find their own ways to cope.

READ MORE IN PENGUIN

PSYCHOLOGY

Introduction to Jung's Psychology Frieda Fordham

'She has delivered a fair and simple account of the main aspects of my psychological work. I am indebted to her for this admirable piece of work' – C. G. Jung in the *Foreword*

Child Care and the Growth of Love John Bowlby

His classic 'summary of evidence of the effects upon children of lack of personal attention … it presents to administrators, social workers, teachers and doctors a reminder of the significance of the family' – *The Times*

Recollections and Reflections Bruno Bettelheim

'A powerful thread runs through Bettelheim's message: his profound belief in the dignity of man, and the importance of seeing and judging other people from their own point of view' – William Harston in the *Independent*. 'These memoirs of a wise old child, candid, evocative, heart-warming, suggest there is hope yet for humanity' – Ray Porter in the *Evening Standard*

Sanity, Madness and the Family R. D. Laing and A. Esterson

Schizophrenia: fact or fiction? Certainly not fact, according to the authors of this controversial book. Suggesting that some forms of madness may be largely social creations, *Sanity, Madness and the Family* demands to be taken very seriously indeed.

I Am Right You Are Wrong Edward de Bono

In this book Dr Edward de Bono puts forward a direct challenge to what he calls the rock logic of Western thinking. Drawing on our understanding of the brain as a self-organizing information system, Dr de Bono shows that perception is the key to more constructive thinking and the serious creativity of design.

READ MORE IN PENGUIN

PSYCHOLOGY

Psychoanalysis and Feminism   Juliet Mitchell

'Juliet Mitchell has risked accusations of apostasy from her fellow feminists. Her book not only challenges orthodox feminism, however; it defies the conventions of social thought in the English-speaking countries … a brave and important book' – *New York Review of Books*

The Divided Self   R. D. Laing

'A study that makes all other works I have read on schizophrenia seem fragmentary … The author brings, through his vision and perception, that particular touch of genius which causes one to say "Yes, I have always known that, why have I never thought of it before?"' – *Journal of Analytical Psychology*

Po: Beyond Yes and No   Edward de Bono

No is the basic tool of the logic system. *Yes* is the basic tool of the belief system. Edward de Bono offers *Po* as a device for changing our ways of thinking: a method for approaching problems in a new and more creative way.

The Informed Heart   Bruno Bettelheim

Bettelheim draws on his experience in concentration camps to illuminate the dangers inherent in all mass societies in this profound and moving masterpiece.

The Care of the Self   Michel Foucault
The History of Sexuality Vol 3

Foucault examines the transformation of sexual discourse from the Hellenistic to the Roman world in an inquiry which 'bristles with provocative insights into the tangled liaison of sex and self' – *The Times Higher Education Supplement*

Mothering Psychoanalysis   Janet Sayers

'An important book … records the immense contribution to psycho-analysis made by its founding mothers' – Julia Neuberger in the *Sunday Times*

READ MORE IN PENGUIN

A CHOICE OF NON-FICTION

Citizens A Chronicle of the French Revolution   Simon Schama

'The most marvellous book I have read about the French Revolution in the last fifty years' – Richard Cobb in *The Times*. 'He has chronicled the vicissitudes of that world with matchless understanding, wisdom, pity and truth, in the pages of this huge and marvellous book' – *Sunday Times*

Out of Africa   Karen Blixen (Isak Dinesen)

Karen Blixen went to Kenya in 1914 to run a coffee-farm; its failure in 1931 caused her to return to Denmark where she wrote this classic account of her experiences. 'A work of sincere power ... a fine lyrical study of life in East Africa' – Harold Nicolson in the *Daily Telegraph*

Yours Etc.   Graham Greene
Letters to the Press 1945–1989

'An entertaining celebration of Graham Greene's lesser-known career as a prolific author of letters to newspapers; you will find unarguable proof of his total addiction to everything about his time, from the greatest issues of the day to the humblest subjects imaginable' – Salman Rushdie in the *Observer*

The Trial of Lady Chatterley   Edited By C. H. Rolph

In October 1960 at the Old Bailey a jury of nine men and three women prepared for the infamous trial of *Lady Chatterley's Lover*. The Obscene Publications Act had been introduced the previous year and D. H. Lawrence's notorious novel was the first to be prosecuted under its provisions. This is the account of the historic trial and acquittal of Penguin Books.

Handbook for the Positive Revolution   Edward de Bono

Edward de Bono's challenging new book provides a practical framework for a serious revolution which has no enemies but seeks to make things better. The hand symbolizes the five basic principles of the Positive Revolution, to remind us that even a small contribution is better than endless criticism.

READ MORE IN PENGUIN

A CHOICE OF NON-FICTION

Riding the Iron Rooster Paul Theroux

Travels in old and new China with the author of *The Great Railway Bazaar*. 'Mr Theroux cannot write badly ... he is endlessly curious about places and people ... and in the course of a year there was almost no train in the whole vast Chinese rail network in which he did not travel' – Ludovic Kennedy

Ninety-two Days Evelyn Waugh

In this fascinating chronicle of a South American journey, Waugh describes the isolated cattle country of Guiana, sparsely populated by an odd collection of visionaries, rogues and ranchers, and records the nightmarish experiences travelling on foot, by horse and by boat through the jungle in Brazil.

The Life of Graham Greene Norman Sherry
Volume One 1904–1939

'Probably the best biography ever of a living author' – Philip French in the *Listener*. Graham Greene has always maintained a discreet distance from his reading public. This volume reconstructs his first thirty-five years to create one of the most revealing literary biographies of the decade.

The Day Gone By Richard Adams

In this enchanting memoir the bestselling author of *Watership Down* tells his life story from his idyllic 1920s childhood spent in Newbury, Berkshire, through public school, Oxford and service in World War Two to his return home and his courtship of the girl he was to marry.

A Turn in the South V. S. Naipaul

'A supremely interesting, even poetic glimpse of a part of America foreigners either neglect or patronize' – *Guardian*. 'An extraordinary panorama' – *Daily Telegraph*. 'A fine book by a fine man, and one to be read with great enjoyment: a book of style, sagacity and wit' – *Sunday Times*

READ MORE IN PENGUIN

A CHOICE OF NON-FICTION

Ginsberg: A Biography Barry Miles

The definitive life of one of this century's most colourful poets. 'A life so dramatic, so dangerous, so committed to hard-volume truth, that his survival is a miracle, his kindness, wisdom and modesty a blessing' – *The Times*. 'Read it to the end' – Michael Horovitz

Coleridge: Early Visions Richard Holmes

'Dazzling … Holmes has not merely reinterpreted Coleridge; he has re-created him, and his biography has the aura of fiction, the shimmer of an authentic portrait … a biography like few I have ever read' –*Guardian*. 'Coleridge lives, and talks and loves … in these pages as never before' – *Independent*

The Speeches of Winston Churchill David Cannadine (ed.)

The most eloquent statesman of his time, Winston Churchill used language as his most powerful weapon. These orations, spanning fifty years, show him gradually honing his rhetoric until, with spectacular effect, 'he mobilized the English language, and sent it into battle'.

Higher than Hope Fatima Meer

A dramatic, personal and intimate biography drawing on letters and reminiscences from Nelson Mandela himself and his close family, *Higher Than Hope* is an important tribute to one of the greatest living figures of our time. It is also a perceptive commentary on the situation in South Africa. No one concerned with politics or humanity can afford to miss it.

Among the Russians Colin Thubron

'The Thubron approach to travelling has an integrity that belongs to another age. And this author's way with words gives his books a value far transcending their topical interest; it is safe to predict that they will be read a century hence' – Dervla Murphy in the *Irish Times*